Alzheimer's
The Answers You Need

by

Helen D. Davies

Michael P. Jensen

ELDER BOOKS
Forest Knolls, California

PRAISE FOR
ALZHEIMER'S: THE ANSWERS YOU NEED

"*Alzheimer's: The Answers You Need* fills an important gap for the person who is developing dementia. It is clear and accessible. The answers are wonderfully sane, practical, and reflect the long experience of the authors. This book will be of value to anyone with a new diagnosis of Alzheimer's and those who care for them."

Nancy Mace, author, The 36 Hour Day

"This book contains encouraging and comforting reminders that there IS life with dementia AND life after diagnosis. Key messages wisely remind readers with Alzheimer's to expect change and to accept necessary help."

Lisa P. Gwyther, MSW
Duke University Medical Center, Durham, NC

"How wonderful to have a book like this available for newly-diagnosed families who need so many answers. This guidebook will be extremely valuable in helping families cope."

Ann Davidson, author, Alzheimer's: A Love Story

"There is no single book which provides so much information in simple language. I recommend this book highly."

Shamala Kanchan, M.D.
Kaiser Permanente, Santa Clara, CA

Library of Congress Cataloging in Publication Data
Main Entry Under Title:
Alzheimer's: The Answers You Need
Davies, Helen D. & Jensen, Michael P.
1. Alzheimer's disease   2. Dementia   3. Self-help   4. Caregiving

ISBN 0-943873-46-0
LCCN 97-060630

Cover Design: Curt Story
Cover Photograph: Stephanie Mohan
Book Design: Bonnie Fisk-Hayden
Printed in the United States of America

THE ALZHEIMER'S BOOKSHELF
PO Box 490 Forest Knolls CA 94933
1 800 909 COPE or 1 415 488 9002
Visit our website on the internet at:
http://www.nbn.com/~elder/alzheimer.html

ELDER BOOKS
Caring for Those Who Care

For all my patients, past and present.

Helen Davies

———⊱◦◦◦⊰———

To Dale Thompson, a gentleman to the end.

Mike Jensen

INTRODUCTION

If you are reading this book, chances are you have Alzheimer's disease, or are trying to help someone who does. You may be feeling depressed, hopeless, and helpless. This book was written to give you help. When you no longer feel helpless, it is easier to deal with depression and hopelessness.

There really *is* help, a lot of help. We will take you step-by-step through the problems most patients face, and tell you the solutions to all the problems that *have* solutions. We will be honest, and tell you when a problem cannot be solved. You may be surprised to find that most problems *do* have solutions. There are ways to cope with most of the changes Alzheimer's disease will force on you during the next few years. These solutions aren't always easy, but they are very real.

The solutions we offer have already worked for many suffering from this disease. They can work for you too. Let us be your companion as you work through these difficult issues.

You may decide to read this book from cover to cover, or you may choose to use the Index to find the subjects that concern you most. The book was written in a question-and-answer format because we have found that is the best way for folks with Alzheimer's disease to take in information. The question-and-answer format also makes that information easier to find. A patient may want to read this book on their own, or have a caregiver read it to them. If you can still read, but have trouble finding the right pages, we suggest your caregiver find the section you want, then let you read the book on your own. *How* you get help doesn't matter. What matters is that you get it.

We know the next few years will not be easy, but they can be a lot better than you think. Please use what you learn here to have the best lives possible.

WHAT IS ALZHEIMER'S DISEASE?

Alzheimer's Disease is a disease of forgetfulness. It causes the connections between brain cells to become ineffective, and the cells themselves to shut down and eventually die. This results in:

- Memory loss

- Personality changes

- Difficulty concentrating

- Impaired decision-making

- Difficulty solving problems

- Loss of ability to perform routine tasks.

It is a disease that gets worse over time. ■

How Do I Know
I Have Alzheimer's Disease?

A diagnosis of Alzheimer's is usually made by giving a patient a series of tests like those you may have recently taken. These tests determine if your memory loss is caused by something other than Alzheimer's disease. When all other possibilities are eliminated, the doctor concludes that you probably have Alzheimer's disease.

This may sound as if the doctor can easily be wrong, but when the correct tests are given by a knowledgeable physician, the Alzheimer's diagnosis is usually right. Doctors now err less than 10-15% of the time when they make an Alzheimer's diagnosis.

Alzheimer's disease can only be confirmed by examining brain tissue, either at autopsy or by brain biopsy. Obviously, an autopsy cannot be done on a living patient. The brain biopsy procedure is dangerous, so it is seldom used to diagnose Alzheimer's disease in this country.

You may have read about other diagnostic tests in the newspapers. These tests are experimental. Their reliability is still being studied by researchers. ∎

AM I GOING CRAZY?

No, you are not going crazy. You are having trouble remembering things.

You do not express yourself as well as you used to.

You may be short-tempered and make mistakes. That is a much different thing than being crazy.

You have a physical illness. You may be forgetful or get confused, but that is not the same as being "crazy." ■

WILL I DIE FROM THIS?

People with Alzheimer's Disease usually die from causes like pneumonia, strokes, heart disease and cancer, just like most other people.

Alzheimer's Disease itself does not kill you, but it may shorten your life span. In its very advanced stages, people become more prone to falls and become bedridden. This increases the likelihood of developing pneumonia or poor circulation, which can be life-threatening.

Staying active and keeping your body in good physical shape is the best way to prolong your life. ■

How Long Will I Live?

No one can tell how long you will live. People with Alzheimer's disease can live 5 to 20 years, or even more. How long you live depends on a number of things, such as:

- how healthy you are

- how active you are

- how well you take care of yourself

- how stable your environment is

- how much stress you feel, or

- how fast the disease progresses.

To explain that last point, Alzheimer's patients can plateau. For varying periods of time, the disease may grow no worse, or get worse very slowly. At other times, it moves more quickly. No one can predict these plateaus.

Alzheimer's disease progresses faster in some patients than in others. Again, no one knows how quickly it will progress in you.

We cannot predict if your life span will be closer to 5 years or 20. If it progresses slowly for you, and you are in good health, stay active, take good care of yourself, reduce stress and have a stable environment, you can have a reasonable expectation of many more interesting and enjoyable years in your life. ■

HOW FAST WILL I GET WORSE?

We do not know. When we talk about the progress of Alzheimer's Disease we mean that it moves slowly through the brain, turning good cells bad. The cells that aren't bad are still good. You need to get the best use from them by exercising the brain. The following tips may not seem to be directly related to the brain, but experience shows that they do make a difference.

Stay in Good Physical Condition.
The disease drains your physical and mental resources. The mind is sharper when the body is healthy. Regular exercise is a great help.

Maintain a Stable Living Environment.
Condition your brain by having a stable and structured living environment. Avoid confusing surroundings.

Be Socially Active.
Give your brain the stimulation of good company in intimate surroundings.

Have a Positive Attitude.
People often give up when they feel negative and depressed. An open and positive attitude is necessary to keep your brain in the best possible shape.

Avoid Stressful Situations.
Your mental energy goes into coping with the stress, not with meeting all your other needs.

We don't know how long it will be before you get worse. We do know that following this advice is your best chance for doing well. ■

WHAT CAUSES ALZHEIMER'S DISEASE?

Alzheimer's disease affects the brain. We know that abnormal protein deposits, called "plaques" and "tangles" form in the brain, but we do not know why this happens. These plaques and tangles are believed to cause brain cells to stop working and eventually die. Scientists all over the world are working to determine why this happens. Some possible risk factors are:

- CHROMOSOMAL ABNORMALITIES. In some cases, the disease seems to be passed from parents to children, but it is not known how widespread this is.

- NEUROTRANSMITTER DEFICIENCIES. Alzheimer's may be caused by a lack of chemicals that the brain needs to stay healthy.

- HEAD INJURIES. Severe head injuries with loss of consciousness, or recurring head injuries, such as severe concussions, may put individuals at higher risk.

- AUTO-IMMUNE ABNORMALITIES. The part of your body that fights disease sometimes makes a mistake and attacks another part of your body, in this case, the brain. One theory is that such a mistake may cause Alzheimer's disease.

- VIRAL INFECTIONS. Alzheimer's may be a virus that moves very slowly.

Many patients wonder if the disease is the result of hardening of the arteries, or emotional stress. These conditions may aggravate Alzheimer's, but they are not thought to cause the disease.

Age and family history are the only well-known and well-understood risk factors for developing Alzheimer's disease. Age does not cause the disease, but the risk of developing it increases as you grow older. The risk is also higher in some families where consecutive generations have had Alzheimer's. It is hard to say whether this represents a hereditary predisposition to the disease itself, a vulnerability to as yet undetermined environmental factors, or a combination of the two.

Neither age nor family history is a guarantee that you will contract or avoid Alzheimer's disease. They merely indicate who is most and least likely at risk to contract it. ■

Is Alzheimer's Disease Contagious?

No, Alzheimer's disease is not contagious. One of the few things we know about it is that you did not get it from anyone and you cannot give it to anyone. You are *not* a danger to your friends or family. ■

Is Alzheimer's Disease Hereditary?

As with so many aspects of the disease, there hasn't been enough time for researchers to answer this question with certainty. It is possible that there are several types of inheritance.

There is a strong indication that Alzheimer's disease is sometimes passed from one generation to the next, with about 25-40% of the relatives of Alzheimer's patients developing the disease. These families are very much in the minority, probably representing fewer than 5% of all Alzheimer's cases.

Most families do not transmit the disease at this high rate and it does not affect each generation in a predictable way. In some families the illness develops before age 50. It does not strike other families until the family members reach their nineties. In other cases there is no predictable pattern at all. Many patients have no family members known to have had Alzheimer's disease.

Researchers now believe that Alzheimer's disease is not caused by a single factor, but by a number of things that interact differently in different people. Genetic factors alone are not usually enough to bring on the disease. Other risk factors may combine with a person's genetic makeup to put them at higher risk of developing Alzheimer's disease.

Unless there is a strong family history of early onset Alzheimer's disease, and it has affected more than one generation, your children should not be too concerned. However, anyone in your family who is exhibiting symptoms typical of the early stages of Alzheimer's should be tested by a doctor. ∎

WILL MY CHILDREN RESENT ME BECAUSE I PUT THEM AT RISK OF GETTING ALZHEIMER'S DISEASE?

It is unlikely your children will resent you for putting them at risk. That would be a very unusual reaction.

The reaction your children will probably have is fear. Since someone so close to them has contracted Alzheimer's disease, they realize they could get it too. They fear for themselves.

This is perfectly natural. It is healthy for them to talk this fear out with a family member, a friend or a counselor. Encourage them to do so. ■

WHAT MISTAKE DID I MAKE
THAT GAVE ME THIS DISEASE?

You did not contract Alzheimer's disease as a result of a mistake you made. So far, only two known factors contribute to developing Alzheimer's disease. They are:

- Age

- A strong family history of Alzheimer's disease.

Both of these are beyond your control. That means that you did nothing to bring it on yourself, and there is nothing you could have done to prevent it. It is not the result of committing some sin. No one gave it to you. The disease just happens as some people get older.

It has been suggested that some environmental or lifestyle factors contribute to contracting Alzheimer's disease. This is under investigation but, so far, nothing outside your own body has been proven to contribute to acquiring the disease. Please do not waste your time and mental energy blaming yourself or anyone else. It is not fair, but Alzheimer's disease just happens. ■

Is There A Treatment Available For Alzheimer's?

There is not yet a definitive treatment for Alzheimer's, but we are hopeful there will be in the future. Don't be fooled by what you hear. The press often announces break-throughs in Alzheimer's research. Progress *is* being made, but these aren't the kinds of break-throughs that give us a sudden cure. It is better to think of each break-through as a piece in a very large jigsaw puzzle. We have more pieces now than we had five years ago, but there are many more pieces yet to find. Researchers may not find a cure for your generation, but they may find one for the next.

There are some experimental drugs being tested, but they do not cure or prevent the disease. The hope is that they can slow the disease's progress. Not all the data is in yet, but some medications seem to retard the progress of Alzheimer's, for a limited period of time, in a very small number of patients. Some patients claim an improved attention span, feel more alert and more motivated when taking these drugs. These are not miraculous changes, but the results are encouraging. Cognex was the first of these drugs approved by the U.S. Food and Drug Administration specifically to treat Alzheimer's disease. Aricept (Donepezil), a second drug, has more recently been approved. Here is a list of some of the drugs now being tested:

- Acetyl -L- Carnitine

- Alzene

- DHEA

- Estrogen

- Ginkgo Biloba

- Milameline

- NGF (Nerve Growth Factor)

- Nimodipine

- Ibuprofen

- Motrin

- Vitamin E

- Selegiline (Eldepryl).

If you want to participate in an experimental drug treatment program you should contact your doctor, your state Alzheimer's Diagnostic & Resource Center, or your local university-affiliated Medical Center. You should also contact the institutions listed in Appendix A. ■

WILL HIGH DOSES OF VITAMINS HELP?

Staying healthy does help, and to do that, you should have the suggested minimum daily amount of vitamins and minerals. Regular nutritious meals will help provide them. If for some reason you cannot get the vitamins you need from food, take a vitamin supplement.

Researchers are studying the effectiveness of anti-oxidants, such as Vitamin E, in slowing the progress of Alzheimer's disease. There is some indication that high doses of Vitamin E may, for a limited period of time, help you when performing everyday activities. It does not improve memory or cognition. High doses of Vitamin E can cause bleeding. The long term affects of high doses of Vitamin E are not yet fully understood.

There is no clear evidence that high doses of any vitamin directly affects Alzheimer's. There is plenty of evidence that high vitamin doses can cause stomach irritation and have other unpleasant side effects. Avoid unnecessary high doses of vitamins, and always check with your doctor before taking any drug or vitamin supplements. ∎

WILL HERBAL REMEDIES HELP?

There is no evidence that herbal remedies help. Some people consider them a valid alternative treatment and want to take them anyway. If that describes you, see your doctor first to make sure you will not have an adverse reaction to the herbal remedy.

Take care to get your herbal medicine from a reliable source. Some herbs have impurities and can become contaminated. ■

WHAT CAN I DO TO HELP MYSELF?

This is one of the most commonly asked questions by Alzheimer's patients. Your activities are limited by the disease. Medications and operations will not halt the progression of Alzheimer's, but you can work to improve the quality of your life in the years to come. There are four major ways to do this:

1. STAY HEALTHY. Alzheimer's disease seems to thrive when a patient becomes ill. Of course, you cannot avoid getting sick, but you can lessen the chances by doing the following:
   - Eat nutritious meals

   - Lose weight, if necessary

   - Do not smoke

   - Have regular check-ups.

2. EXERCISE. A research project which studied two groups of A.D. patients demonstrated the benefits of exercise. One group had a half-hour conversation everyday, while the other group went for a half-hour walk. The results of this study showed that the group that walked did better than the group that talked.

We recommend:
- WALKING EXERCISE. Walking is good for the whole body and especially good for helping patients keep their walking coordination. Alzheimer's disease diminishes walking coordination, so walking exercise is very help-ful. Make it a habit to go for a half-hour walk daily.

- TAI-CHI. Research shows that older adults benefit from practicing Tai-Chi. It improves balance, so patients are less likely to accidentally fall. It can be done in a group, and that will increase your social contacts.

- **OTHER EXERCISE.** Consult your doctor first, then choose what you like to do. Consider calisthenics, swimming, running, bicycling with a friend, or using a stationary bicycle or a rowing machine. It is important to get your heart rate up for a few minutes every day. Exercise, along with walking, helps you stay strong and in good health.

3. **MENTAL STIMULATION.** Alzheimer's disease dulls your mind. The following are steps you can take to keep the unaffected cells active:
   - Invite guests in
   - Accept invitations out
   - Attend movies, concerts and other cultural activities or sports events
   - Join an Alzheimer's support group
   - See nature in the wild, or at the zoo
   - Travel
   - Write or tape record your life story.

4. **POSITIVE ATTITUDE.** *Do not give up.* Find new ways to do anything that is difficult for you. For example,
   - If you lose your job, do volunteer work
   - If you can't drive, think of other things that will be fun for both you and your caregiver
   - If you cannot read, listen to tapes, enjoy art books, books of photography, or family pictures
   - Do not be afraid to try and fail
   - Do not feel sorry for yourself
   - Do not be embarrassed to have Alzheimer's
   - Discuss Alzheimer's openly with family and friends.

We don't have a cure for Alzheimer's disease, but we can work with you, your family, and friends to give you the best and most highly functioning life possible. The goal is to keep you healthy, stress-free, and functioning at your maximum capacity. ∎

AM I DOING EVERYTHING I CAN TO HELP MYSELF?

When you have an illness that has no specific treatment, it is natural to wonder if you can do more. Ask yourself these questions:

- Have you had a thorough evaluation by a knowledgeable physician?

- Are you taking care of your physical health?

- If you are depressed, are you receiving help to deal with your feelings?

- Are you keeping as active as possible?

- Are you taking advantage of services that are available to you?

- Are you and your family keeping abreast of new information about Alzheimer's disease. (The Alzheimer's Association provides an excellent newsletter.)

- Have you considered participating in a research program?

- Do you and your family attend an Alzheimer's support group?

- Are you keeping down your level of stress?

If you answered yes, then you are doing everything you can to help yourself.

If your answer is no, then use the list above to help you help yourself. ■

How Can I Find Out More About This Disease?

Most of the information about Alzheimer's disease is written in such a way that a patient will have trouble finding and understanding what they want to know. There is, however, much good material that will be helpful to your caregiver. If you can still read without becoming frustrated, you should try to read up on the disease. You can watch video tapes about the disease if reading has become too difficult. Your local State Department of Health and your local library will be able to provide more information. You can also request a list of materials from these two organizations:

Alzheimer's Association
191 North Michigan Ave, Suite 1000
Chicago IL 60611-1676   1-800-272-3900

ADEAR Center
P. O. Box 8250
Silver Spring MD 20907-8250   1-800-438-4380

WHAT IS A CAREGIVER?

The word 'caregiver' practically defines itself. A caregiver is one who gives care, but it has a particular application to one caring for an Alzheimer's patient.

Alzheimer's disease makes you progressively less able to do things that you were once able to do. Your caregiver is the person who helps you to do those things. Someday, you will no longer be able to drive. Your caregiver will drive you. Someday, you will have trouble remembering appointments. Your caregiver will remind you. Whether you need a little help, or a lot of help, your caregiver is there to help.

A caregiver is usually your spouse. Your spouse probably lives with you, and is in the best position to give care. However, a caregiver can be anyone — a son or daughter, another relative, a friend, or someone hired to help you. ■

What Is Meant By A Structured Life?

Leading a structured life means that you stick to a regular routine in familiar places. Since most people diagnosed with Alzheimer's cannot work at regular jobs, they cannot benefit from the structure that comes with having a job. You and your caregiver need to sit down and develop a structure that works for both of you. It should include:

- Where you spend your days

- How you spend your time

- The kind of exercise you do

- Time spent away from home

- Time spent with other people.

The familiar should be part of your routine. You may get confused in unfamiliar surroundings and with unfamiliar people. It is therefore good to spend time at home and in the homes of friends. Adult daycare is very good, but you must attend often enough so that it becomes familiar. We recommend going to daycare at least two or three days a week. Patients do better when this structure is part of a regular routine.

When you spend time alone at home, it is helpful if your caregiver leaves a written itinerary of the day's activities. There is an example on the next page. This itinerary helps you spend your time usefully and suggests what you can do next, should you have trouble remembering. ■

SCHEDULE FOR TODAY'S ACTIVITIES

Good morning! *It is Friday, July 18th, 1998.*

Don't forget to put on your watch.

There is a bowl of cereal on the kitchen table and milk in the refrigerator.

After breakfast, you might enjoy recording your autobiography for the kids. I left the tape recorder on the kitchen table. The tape is ready to go. Just press the Record button.

10 A.M.   I'll call to see how you're doing.

11 A.M.   Ray will come by to take you for a walk.

12:30 P.M. Have lunch. There is a sandwich and napkin in the orange Tupperware container in the fridge.

After lunch, you can listen to the radio. I set the radio dial to your favorite station.

2.00 P.M.   I'll call again. After I call, why not turn on the TV set?

5.20 P.M.   I will arrive home.

6.30 P.M.   We will go to Ethel and Evan's for dinner. ∎

WHY AM I TAKING ALL THESE TESTS?

The first tests you took were used as diagnostic tools. They were a way to find out if your memory loss was caused by Alzheimer's disease or something else. Since the progression of Alzheimer's cannot be physically measured, these tests continue. It is like having a check-up for your mind. The tests reveal your strengths and weaknesses; they indicate how you are doing. ■

How Are These Tests Going To Help Me?

The tests help you in two ways:

- They confirm that you have Alzheimer's disease. Memory loss caused by something else may be treatable. If the results show that you do not have Alzheimer's, other measures can be taken.

- It is in your best interest to have you, your doctor, and your family informed of the progress of the disease. How far has it gone? What can you expect next? How should you prepare for the future? What changes should you make now? The test results will point out your strengths and weaknesses. With this knowledge, you can plan ways to use your strengths to compensate for those areas in which you have trouble. ■

WHY DO THEY ASK ME
THE SAME QUESTIONS AGAIN AND AGAIN?

The reason for repeating questions is to get accurate results. Alzheimer's disease causes memory loss and the questions test your memory.

Let's say they test you five times by asking you the same question. You know the answer the first two times, but not the next three. That indicates a memory loss. Different questions would not adequately test your memory, since each memory would only be tested once.

Your answers are combined with the answers to other questions, and those answers are checked over time. Only by asking the same questions again and again can your test results be accurately compared to your previous tests. ■

WILL THE TEST RESULTS BE PRACTICAL?

Every patient's experience is unique. Alzheimer's disease progresses at different speeds and in patterns that are not strictly predictable. Some patients may have their visual/spatial perception affected quite early, while others may not be affected in this area until later. Some have early trouble with numbers, while others can do math for a comparatively long time.

These tests let you and your doctor know how you are doing. They reveal your mental *strengths* and *weaknesses*. They can help you live a better life. Here are two examples of how you can live better by knowing your *strengths*:

- You may be able to understand written cues better than spoken cues. The tests will reveal this. Your doctor can then suggest that your caregiver use written lists or drawings to improve communication with you.

- Perhaps you like reading, but now find reading difficult. Good results on your visual/spatial tests suggest that you can still have fun with your leisure time by doing puzzles, or by playing cards or board games. If your past memory is good, you can tape-record your autobiography and pass down your life-story to future generations.

Here are two examples of how you can live better by knowing your *weaknesses*:

- If you are still driving, but test poorly in visual/spatial perception, that tells you it is time to *stop driving before you have an accident.*

- If you are still doing your own finances, but have trouble with numbers, that tells you *it is time to turn your finances over to someone else before you bounce a check.*

Knowing your strengths and weaknesses helps to enrich your life. It can guide you and your caregiver in developing techniques that will help you live more easily and avoid the frustration that comes with mistakes. ∎

I Want To Know More
About Drug-Testing Programs

Discuss your interest in drug-testing programs with your physician. Your doctor can make referrals. You can also obtain a list of centers that conduct drug studies from the Alzheimer's Association.

You must understand that these drugs are not miracle cures. *They may not be helpful.* The results, so far, are mixed. The progress of the disease appears to have slowed somewhat in some patients who have participated in drug-testing programs. A minority of them show a small amount of improvement. The earlier you begin drug treatment, the longer you can function comparatively well. It is a good idea to participate in a drug program. That way you will do everything you can for yourself, and you will help researchers stop Alzheimer's disease.

Research drugs are studied under very strict criteria. The criteria vary from study to study, but generally you will find:

- Half the patients take the real drug, and half take a placebo. You will not know which you received until the study is over.

- Many studies allow the patient to take the actual drug after the test period is over. You still take it under research conditions, but you will now know you are not receiving a placebo.

- Each study has its own eligibility criteria. You must meet these criteria to participate. They usually require you be in good physical health and complete a specified level of cognitive testing.

We want to encourage you to seriously consider participating in a drug program. The knowledge that you are doing everything you can, not only for yourself, but to end Alzheimer's disease, can give you a real boost. ∎

WHY SHOULD I PARTICIPATE
IN A DRUG RESEARCH PROGRAM?

There are three reasons why you should consider participating in a drug research program:

- The more research that is done, the sooner a cure, control or preventive for Alzheimer's will be developed. You can help that process.

- While the drugs do not seem to help most people afflicted with Alzheimer's, some patients do report feeling mentally sharper. If the drugs help *them*, they may also help *you*.

- Most patients get a tremendous psychological boost when they do everything they can to fight the effects of Alzheimer's disease. A drug research program is one more way you can assert yourself against Alzheimer's disease. By helping to beat Alzheimer's, you help your children and all future generations who may face this disease. ■

Can I Continue To Work?

Whether or not you can continue to work depends on the degree of your impairment and the demands of your job. A diagnosis of Alzheimer's disease will usually make it impossible for you to perform work that requires complex decisions or skilled tasks. It will also impair your ability to learn new information and meet deadlines.

You may continue to work if:

- Your employer knows you have Alzheimer's disease and feels comfortable employing you.

- The work requires structured, repetitive tasks or manual activity.

Many patients find that volunteer work is best. They can help others without the pressure of a disapproving boss. Volunteers also have flexibility in the number of hours and days of the week that they work. As the degree of your impairment grows, you will no longer be able to adequately perform your job, and will need to retire. Staying active with a job or volunteer work is one of the best ways of keeping sharp that part of your mind not affected by Alzheimer's disease. ∎

How Much Longer
Can I Hold On To My Job?

How much longer you can hold on to your job depends on a number of things:

1. THE TYPE OF JOB YOU HAVE. Activities like meeting deadlines, making critical decisions, learning new information, high-tech work, or anything highly skilled will become very difficult. If your job involves any of these, you will need to retire. If you have a low skill, non-technical position, you may be able to continue for some time. How long you stay is determined by how quickly Alzheimer's affects you.

2. HOW MUCH THE DISEASE HAS DEVELOPED. Some patients do not know they have a problem until the disease affects their job performance. They go to their doctor to learn the cause of their problems at work, and then discover they have Alzheimer's. At that point, it is difficult for them to keep their job.

3. IT DEPENDS ON THE TOLERANCE OF YOUR EMPLOYER. Everyone makes mistakes at work, but Alzheimer's patients are more prone to mistakes than others. Any intelligent employer tolerates a certain number of mistakes, knowing that to err is human. In time, Alzheimer's patients will make an intolerable number of mistakes, and lose their jobs if they do not retire on their own.

4. IT DEPENDS ON THE ACCEPTANCE OF YOUR CO-WORKERS. Having a person affected by Alzheimer in the workplace is potentially disruptive for two reasons:

   • Many people are not psychologically secure enough to be comfortable when someone has a disease as serious as Alzheimer's. They can divide a workplace between those who support you and those who wish you were not there.

- As time passes, the number of mistakes you make will increase. Some co-workers may not trust your judgment. Again, a workplace can become divided between those who are supportive and those who resent what they feel is special treatment.

We hope your workplace is full of tolerant and supportive people who can cope with your illness. Of course, your employer cannot tolerate a serious division in the work force. Should you, through no fault of your own, cause such a division, there is a good chance you will be let go.

You also need to consider the financial impact on you. Weigh the pros and cons of taking disability, or early retirement as opposed to severance pay. You will need to give up your job eventually. It makes sense to get the best financial package you can. ■

SHOULD I TELL MY CO-WORKERS THAT I HAVE ALZHEIMER'S?

The decision to tell your co-workers about your diagnosis depends on how closely you interact with them and how much difficulty you have doing your job. If you make mistakes or cannot keep up, your co-workers will become frustrated with you. Then it is best to discuss the situation with the co-workers closest to you. What you tell them will depend on:

- Whether you have discussed the problem with your employers, and how they feel about it

- If your work environment is supportive

- How comfortable you feel about discussing your problem.

At the very least, it is helpful to acknowledge that there is a problem and that you are seeking medical help to deal with it. It is not always necessary to discuss the diagnosis with everyone. It may suffice to say that you have a neurological disorder that affects your memory. The more comfortable you are telling co-workers, the better off you will be. Co-workers can be helpful when they understand the problem and how they can help you. ■

How Can I Have Self-Esteem Now That I Do Not Have A Job?

Many people think their self-esteem depends on their job, or on their ability to work. That is a mistake.

Many people who have jobs also have a problem with self-esteem. *A job is only a part of our lives.* It gives us an income, companionship, and a way to structure our lives. Most people have some degree of insecurity in their positions. They are unhappy when they displease their employers. That is not self-worth.

For self-esteem to last, it must come from within. Anything outside should not affect it. A job is outside of us. If you base your self-esteem on your job, and then lose your job, you also lose your self-esteem. It makes more sense to base self-worth on your own character. Then your self-esteem will remain intact no matter what happens to you.

Real Self-Worth

Following is a list of personal characteristics you can base your self-worth upon. Feel free to add your own personal qualities. For example, you are:

- A loving, gracious, generous person
- A loyal friend
- A giving spouse
- A caring parent
- Loved by those who you love.

Here are some things you can do to increase your self-esteem:

- Help others

- Participate in Alzheimer's research

- Remember that you have had success in your life.

If you lost your job (and your self-worth with it), we sympathize. We also suggest that you begin building self-esteem from the inside. The more secure you are, the better equipped you will be emotionally to deal with all aspects of Alzheimer's disease. Counseling can be a great help, so do not hesitate to see a counselor.

While it is true that you can no longer do many things that were once easy, you can still provide love and affection to your family and friends. You can still help others who are less fortunate than you. You can choose to participate in research that may help discover the cause and a possible treatment for Alzheimer's disease.

The important thing is not to get caught in the trap of thinking, *I can no longer work; therefore, I am worthless.* ■

May I Still Drink Alcohol?

It is best to abstain from alcohol. An *occasional* glass of wine or beer is probably all right, but anything more is not.

As people grow older, they do not tolerate alcohol well, and metabolize it less efficiently. This is even more acute in Alzheimer's patients. Patients often feel confused. Alcohol adds to that confusion. It also puts an extra burden on the body and causes brain cell damage. Practically speaking, alcohol and Alzheimer's do not mix. ■

CAN I CONTINUE TO HANDLE CASH?

This question does not have a yes-or-no answer. Alzheimer's disease will slowly take away your ability to handle money. You probably *can* handle money for a while but, in time, it will become difficult to figure out the right amount needed to make a purchase. You will also have trouble knowing if you received the correct change. Some patients forget to put their money away, they hold it in their hands, which is dangerous in some neighborhoods.

It is our theme in this book that if you *can* do something, you *should*. If you can only do a part, do that part, and get help with the rest. If you can no longer do something, let it go, and concentrate on what you *can* do. It is the same for handling money. When you have trouble figuring out what to pay for a purchase, or counting your change, then only handle money when your caregiver is around. Should you then need help, it will be there. ■

Should I Continue To Handle My Finances?

Some patients can handle their finances, and some cannot. All Alzheimer's patients need help eventually. You not only need the math skills to add, subtract, and do percentages, you need to remember to pay bills on time and to balance the checkbook. It is also difficult to make investment decisions.

Alzheimer's disease will someday compromise your ability to do all of this. It may have already begun to affect you. If you *can* handle your finances for now, you *should*.

Always have your caregiver review what you do. It is easy to make a financial mistake, and those mistakes can be very costly. Did you add the numbers correctly? Are there any bills that you missed? Are there any checks you forgot to deposit? Your caregiver will catch these things.

Patients have had their power shut off and their phones disconnected because they simply forgot the first, second, and third notices. Please do not let that happen to you. Make sure everything is double-checked.

Another problem is the possibility of strangers taking advantage of you. This happened to a woman we know. When her neighbors found out she had Alzheimer's disease, they came by her house everyday, asking for money. In her confusion, she forgot they had been there the day before. They even tried to get her to go to her bank with them to withdraw her savings. Thank goodness she could not remember where she put her bank book, and that her son found out what was happening.

Patients are simply not equipped to handle scam artists. Keep your caregiver involved in all financial transactions to reduce this risk. ■

MAY I STILL SMOKE?

We urge you to give up smoking. If the health hazard to you and those with whom you live does not motivate you to stop, consider this: *Your new forgetfulness creates a fire hazard, as well.* Most fires in the home are caused by smokers who neglect a burning cigarette through sleep or forgetfulness. Someone with Alzheimer's disease is far more likely to forget a burning cigarette than someone without the disease. For this reason, as well as the other health risks involved, we urge you to give up smoking now. ■

WILL I BECOME VIOLENT?

You will probably not become violent. Fewer than 10% of Alzheimer's patients do. If it happens, it will be when the disease has progressed.

You may still be worried. What if you are among that 10% of patients who become violent?

When a patient becomes violent, it is usually the response to a confusing environment. They may be in an unfamiliar place or in a crowded room. They feel something is demanded of them, but do not know how to respond. It is usually under these circumstances that a patient strikes out, and the reason is frustration.

If an Alzheimer's patient becomes violent, it is not because they are bad people; it is because they are afraid. A smart caregiver will avoid situations that may result in violence.

The reasons you should feel hopeful are:

- Most Alzheimer's patients never become violent

- Medication can control violent tendencies

- For most who *do* become violent, it is just a phase— it will pass. ■

WILL I BECOME INCONTINENT?

Incontinence means losing control of your bladder or bowel. Bladder incontinence is a common problem for many older adults, not just Alzheimer's patients. In the late stage of the disease, bowel incontinence also becomes a problem. Alzheimer's disease causes incontinence in two ways:

- The disease affects the brain's control over all bodily functions, including the muscles that constrain the bladder and bowel.

- The memory loss and lack of coordination caused by Alzheimer's can make the bathroom hard to find. Clothes become difficult to remove in time.

A patient may have incontinence not caused by Alzheimer's disease. It can be caused by other health problems, like infection or a reaction to drugs, or even an emotional reaction. The most common cause of bladder incontinence in women is stress. Bladder incontinence occurs when you laugh or cough. These forms of incontinence usually respond to treatment.

Your doctor can assess the cause of incontinence and make recommendations that will help deal with this problem. ■

Will They Take My Driver's License Away?

Yes, your drivers license will eventually be taken away. The question is *when*, and that depends on two things:

- The specific areas of memory and cognition affected by the disease

- What stage the disease has reached.

The only way to know if you should drive is to undergo testing. Tests are conducted by your local Department of Motor Vehicles or by specialized outside agencies. Many states have laws requiring doctors to report Alzheimer's cases, and those states usually require you to take a driving test. You do not want to injure yourself or anyone else because you are driving when you should not be. *If you have Alzheimer's Disease, please do not drive until you have been tested.*

Even if you are allowed to keep your license for a time, you could become a dangerous driver without realizing it. You may also lose your ability to recognize landmarks. If your caregiver asks you to stop driving, trust them, and stop. Due to the effects of Alzheimer's Disease, your caregiver is now a better judge of your driving ability than you are.

Of course, you can still use your car for transportation, and to take trips, but it is best to turn the driving over to someone else. ■

Why Won't They Let Me Drive?

One of the most traumatic issues for an Alzheimer's patient is not being allowed to drive.

Patients are no longer good judges of their own driving abilities. Perhaps you remember the mechanics of driving a car, and believe that you can handle any driving situation as well as you did in the past. *This is the disease fooling you.* Research shows that people with Alzheimer's disease are five times more likely to have an accident than others their age without memory problems. In one study, nearly half of all Alzheimer's drivers had an accident.

Patients who drive have disappeared for days and not remembered where they were. They do not notice every stop sign and red light. They have poor judgment in dangerous situations. Their reaction time is slower in an emergency. Their hand/eye coordination suffers, and so does the way they see the relationships between objects.

You may have been a great driver all your life. You may never have had an accident, or even a ticket. But you now have Alzheimer's disease, and that makes all the difference. Everyone with Alzheimer's disease is a bad driver. The longer you have the disease, the worse your driving will become. A car is a lethal weapon, too dangerous to trust to someone who is not functioning at their best, and no Alzheimer's patient is functioning at their best. That is why they will not let you drive. ∎

What Should I Do
If I Am Out Driving And Get Lost?

You *will* get lost someday. All Alzheimer's patients who drive eventually *do* get lost. Be prepared. Refer to the check list below to help you deal with this situation when it happens. Copy the checklist, or cut it out of this book and put it in your car, so you will always have it with you when driving. Do not put it in the glove compartment, or you may forget it is there. We suggest taping it to the dashboard, where it will always be visible.

Driver's Checklist

Never leave your house without:

- A card listing your name, address, and phone number. Keep the card in your pocket or wallet. It is a good idea to include a note saying you have Alzheimer's disease, and asking anyone who reads it to help you.

- A Safe Return bracelet from the Alzheimer's Association or a Medic Alert bracelet for Alzheimer's disease.

- Enough change to make some long-distance phone calls.

If you do get lost:

- Only drive as far as the next building or business. *Do not keep driving.* You will end up even further from home.

- Stop at that building, and park.

- Ask someone to help you.

- Do not ask for directions and try to drive back home. If you got lost once, you probably will again.

- If you have a car-phone, dial 911.

- Do not phone home yourself. You do not know where you are. Your caregiver cannot help unless someone tells them where to find you. Ask for help. Have a local person make the call for you, since they know where you are. They can give your caregiver directions. If they cannot reach your caregiver, they can call the police to help.

IF YOU DO NOT SEE ANY BUILDINGS:

- Pull to the side of the road, raise the hood of the car, put on your emergency flashers. Do not leave the car. Wait for someone to stop. If you have a handkerchief or scarf, tie it to your antenna. This will tell passersby that you need help.

IF YOU CANNOT TELL ANYONE THE INFORMATION THEY NEED
TO HELP YOU:

- Show them the note which lists your name, address, and phone number and states that you have Alzheimer's disease.

- Point to your Medic Alert bracelet or your Safe Return bracelet. ■

What Should I Do
If I Am Out Walking And Get Lost?

- **Stay Calm.** A person who panics cannot solve this problem.

- **Sit down.** Wait for your panic to pass, and organize your thoughts.

- **Do Not Keep Going.** You may be going in the wrong direction.

OK, you are now calm. What next? You are alone. You do not know the way home. You cannot remember your home address, and you do not recognize where you are. What do you do?

- **Always wear an ID bracelet linked to a 24-hour service.** This will provide full information in case of emergency. Then you will have that information everywhere you go.

- **Never be afraid or embarrassed to ask for help, even from a stranger.** You may be surprised at how helpful a stranger will be if you say you have Alzheimer's and ask for help. They can take you home, call your home, or call the police to help you. Everybody needs a little help sometimes, so do not be afraid or embarrassed to ask.

If you ask someone for help but the words will not come:

- **Show them your ID bracelet.** Tell them what you can about your problem. Most people are clever enough to piece it together. ■

SHOULD I WEAR AN ID BRACELET?

It is an excellent idea to wear an ID bracelet. You must take the possibility of getting lost very seriously. It can happen to any patient, even those who have never been lost. Think of wearing an ID bracelet as an insurance policy with these three benefits:

- Wearing an ID bracelet is the best way to ensure that you get back home.

- The bracelet can alert people to any medical problems you may have.

- Your family will feel better because they will worry less. ■

How Will My Diagnosis Affect My Family?

Having a serious disease is a family problem. It affects everyone who loves you. The way it affects them will depend on the kind of people they are.

Family members who cannot cope with Alzheimer's disease will try to avoid confronting it. You may not see them very often. Those who have a caring and generous nature will become available to help you whenever you need help. You could end up spending more time with your family than you did before. We know of one father and son who saw each other mostly on birthdays and holidays. When the father retired after contracting Alzheimer's disease, they had lunch together every week.

Alzheimer's disease can bring people closer together. When patients openly share their feelings about the disease, and the family members do the same with one another, Alzheimer's disease becomes an opportunity for real closeness. As family members help one another in practical and emotional ways, close ties develop.

Some patients make it hard for themselves and their families by denying to themselves they have Alzheimer's, or pretending to others they do not have it. This robs you of that closeness, and makes everyone's relationship with you dishonest, since they know you have Alzheimer's but feel pressured by you to help cover it up.

Alzheimer's disease can have another unfortunate effect on your family. Some patients falsely accuse their families of conspiring against them or of stealing from them. They get stubborn and will not accept decisions that are in their best interest. Others say angry and hateful things to their families. This puts an emotional strain on everyone.

The key is to establish open and honest communication between you and your family. It is difficult enough to have Alzheimer's disease without the added barriers that come with dishonesty. Having Alzheimer's gives you an opportunity to forge a long-lasting family bond. ∎

I Used To Be The Boss. Now My Spouse Has Taken Over, And I Resent It!

Alzheimer's disease is changing your life. It renders you unable to do everyday things well. Since the disease is progressive, you will someday not be able to do them at all. This includes activities like driving a car, making financial decisions, even getting dressed. The disease works in such a way that you *think* you can do something even after you no longer can. That is why Alzheimer's patients make so many mistakes, and some mistakes are very costly indeed.

Those who love you do not want you to get hurt, nor do they want to see you make mistakes. When they realize you are no longer able to do something for yourself, they naturally want to save you from the frustration, embarrassment and consequences of your failures. This is why they tell you not to drive anymore. It is the reason they take over your finances. It is also why they want you to sign a durable power of attorney or a living trust. They can see the dangers to which Alzheimer's has blinded you.

It is normal for patients to become angry and resentful when this happens. Another function of the disease is that many patients have trouble rising above their resentment. Most can rise above it, at least some of the time. When you feel resentful, try to remember that your loved ones are acting in your best interests, and make the best of it. ■

53

How Will Alzheimer's Disease Change My Marriage?

It is the nature of Alzheimer's disease to make a person more dependent. As your memory and other faculties fade, you will need more help from others. It is natural that help will come from the people who live with you. This greater dependency is at the heart of how your marriage will change.

Does this bother you? No one wants to be a burden to someone they love. Try to think of it like this: If your spouse had Alzheimer's disease, wouldn't you willingly accept that responsibility? Of course you would. You need to let your spouse accept that responsibility for you.

It is particularly hard for men with Alzheimer's disease to accept being dependent. From an early age, society cast them in the roles of leader and financial supporter. Now Alzheimer's disease forces them and their wives to reverse roles. Many men have trouble adjusting to this. Some never do. They blame their wives for taking their role away from them, but this is misplaced anger. Their wives have not taken their role away; the disease has. The wife is just helping to do what the patient cannot do for himself.

This is a problem for women, as well. They resent their husbands taking over responsibilities that have always been theirs, such as cooking and managing the house. A common trap for Alzheimer's patients is to resent spouses who assume more responsibility. It is important for you to accept that you are no longer as able as you once were and to allow your spouse to help. It is also important that you continue to try to do things for yourself. If you *can* do something, you *should*. When you need help, your spouse should help.

It is here that friction comes into the marriage of an

Alzheimer's patient. Sometimes spouses help too much, treating patients as more helpless than they are. Patients understandably resent this. At other times, patients need more help than they are willing to admit, and wrongly resent the spouse. As these problems arise, you need honest, non-angry conversations to overcome them. Counseling has helped some patients and their spouses make these transitions.

Discuss when you need help and what you can still do. Your spouse needs to remember that you are probably more capable than you seem. You need to remember that you are probably less capable than you think you are. Look for solutions you can both live with. ■

HOW WILL MY SPOUSE FEEL ABOUT ME NOW THAT I AM CHANGING?

It is natural to feel concerned that your spouse may not love you or want to stay with you. If you are worried, talk about it. It is better to know than to fret.

You should believe them when they tell you the disease does not change their commitment to you. Most couples stick together. Many couples report growing even closer to one another. One patient actually said, "I had to get sick to bring us together."

Do not forget that spouses struggle with Alzheimer's disease in their own way. They feel frustrated and angry. They may be short-tempered with you. They are really angry at what has happened to you and frustrated that they are powerless to stop it. This does not mean they no longer care for you. To the contrary, if they did not care, it would not affect them.

Our advice is: believe they are still committed to you and enjoy the closeness that a time of trial can bring. ■

I'm Afraid My Spouse Will Leave Me
If I Express My Anger.

Let's distinguish between the two types of anger patients typically feel:

1. **Anger at Having Alzheimer's Disease.** All patients feel this anger. Your husband or wife also feels it. They are angry that you have the disease. Encourage them to talk about their feelings, and they will understand when you do the same. Hiding your feelings increases your anger. It is much better for you both to talk about your feelings than to hide them. The two of you have a chance to help each other by discussing your anger as openly as you can.

2. **Anger at your Caregiver.** This part is scary, because to talk about it is to risk chasing your caregiver away. You might, if your intention is just to tell them off. However, there is a way of doing it that can bring you closer. Both of you need to speak, not in anger, but to explain what makes you angry. This lets your caregiver know how to behave differently and gives you some control over the way you are treated. You will have less anger because your caregiver will treat you better. It takes two people with the right attitude to make this work. Talking with a counselor can help.

It is easier not to say anything and keep your anger to yourself, but that will not work. You will just grow angrier until you snap and say something that is cruel and destructive. Patients often do this. It is better to talk and grow closer than to stay silent and grow further apart. ■

How Will Alzheimer's Change My Sex Life?

There are five things to understand about the sexuality of an Alzheimer's patient:

1. Your need to be physically close to another person will not change. Everybody needs affection, whether it be holding hands, hugging, or actual intercourse.

2. Some men experience impotency during the early stages of Alzheimer's disease. If this happens, see your doctor. Many patients are helped by professional treatment.

3. Because Alzheimer's disease affects your memory, you may need to be led by your partner. You may enjoy what you are doing, but forget the next step. Your partner can lead you out of this difficulty. This can become a problem if you have always had the role of initiator in your sex play. You may not like their help. Try to remember the effect of the disease, and welcome this help as a benefit to both of you.

4. One way Alzheimer's disease affects memory is to make a patient forget they had intercourse shortly after completing it. Your partner, who does not have a memory problem, may not be as keen to have intercourse again. Try not to feel rejected or lied to when your partner refuses for this reason.

5. Male caregivers often feel they are taking unfair sexual advantage when their mates have Alzheimer's disease, even when their partner indicates a willingness for sex play. That is understandable and their sensitivity is commendable. We suggest taking it slowly. If your partner is willing, she will respond. If she does not respond, you know she is not willing. ■

Will My Teenage Children
Have Special Problems?

Your teenage children probably *will* have special problems. The teenage years are a time when children establish their own identity, separate from their family identity. They usually find part of their identity with their peer group. A teenager who has a parent with Alzheimer's disease may feel embarrassed and different from these peers. Since the disease is changing the dynamics of their family, and they do not feel part of their peer group, they do not feel as if they belong anywhere.

There is a sense of losing both parents, as well. As the disease progresses, patients are less able to care for their children. As spouses become caregivers, they become less available to the rest of their families, leaving their children somewhat on their own. The teenager typically feels great anger, and seldom knows how to deal with that. *Counseling is recommended.*

Alzheimer's disease is very expensive. This has prevented some children from going to college, which is also expensive.

A special problem arises when the father of a teenage son develops Alzheimer's disease. When sons take on their father's responsibilities, the father often becomes resentful. His pride is already undermined by the disease, and the role reversal is too much for many men to take; some have even threatened their sons. This makes the son feel guilty. With all the tension in the house and potential embarrassment over the father's behavior, these boys may not want to bring their friends home and may not like to be at home themselves. They often withdraw, do poorly in school, or get into trouble. Some turn to drugs. A number have attempted suicide. It helps when children find a surrogate as a role model.

How well things go depends largely on how good the family dynamics were before the disease. The healthier the family environment, the better off you will all be.

You cannot avoid the strain on your teenage children. By understanding the cause of this strain, you and your caregiver will be in the best position to handle it. The following guidelines will help you to minimize family stress:

- Get counseling for your teenagers

- Consider counseling for your entire family

- Prepare for the future financial burden well in advance

- Allow your teenagers to develop a surrogate relationship with someone else

- Encourage your teenagers to bring their friends home and to be open with their friends about your disease

- Try not to resent your teenager taking over a responsibility you once had — they are only trying to help. ■

SHOULD WE TELL OUR FRIENDS?

Yes, it is to everyone's advantage if you do. Since Alzheimer's will make you search for words, forget information, and make mistakes, your friends will see that something is wrong anyway. It makes sense to explain your new behaviors by telling your friends you have Alzheimer's. This allows you to ask for help when Alzheimer's stymies you. It will set many of your friends at ease when they understand the cause of your new behavior.

Simply explain what Alzheimer's is and the effect it is having on you. Tell them what you would like from them as friends. For example, tell your friends when you would like help and when you would not. Assure them that even though Alzheimer's will change your life, you want to keep it normal for as long as you can, so you want to keep your friendship intact.

This continued social contact is very good for an Alzheimer's patient. Continue to enjoy your friends just as before, but make it easier on everyone by talking openly about Alzheimer's disease. ■

WILL MY FRIENDS REJECT ME?

This question does not have a simple yes-or-no answer. It is a complex problem that starts with the disease. You may have trouble following a conversation. You may lose your place while telling a story. Your friends will notice these changes. They can respond in two ways:

- Some will take it in stride and try to help

- Others will feel uncomfortable or react in fear.

Some people fear disease so much that they cannot bear to see it. They may let your friendship cool. This is not because they reject you, or because they are bad people; they simply are not strong enough to bear with you. Many patients grow bitter about such friends. Bitterness will not help. Try to remember that your friends are not rejecting you, they are reacting in fear.

Many will seize the opportunity to prove their friendship. They will continue to spend time with you. Whenever you need help, they will be available. Alzheimer's disease thus becomes a way to show just how deep some friendships can be. ■

WHAT IS THE BEST ATTITUDE TO HAVE?

The best attitude to have is what we call an "open and positive" attitude. Some patients dwell on their limitations, rather than on their possibilities. They get stuck at the "why me?" stage and feel sorry for themselves.

The period between the first symptoms and the more severe manifestations of Alzheimer's can be ten years or more. There are many years in which you can remain active and enjoy life. An open and positive attitude keeps you open to new possibilities. Alzheimer's disease may limit you but, within those limits, you can redefine your life in a positive way. The rest of this section presents suggestions for steps you can take to live as fully as possible. A patient with the wrong attitude will *not* do these things. A patient with the best attitude *will*.

Begin by expressing your sadness and anger over contracting Alzheimer's, then seek the support of your family and friends. This does not imply you will pity yourself or get others to feel sorry for you. Rather, acknowledging and expressing your feelings is a way of progressing beyond them.

Once you are over that initial anger, take care of the legal issues that all Alzheimer's patients must attend to. Draw up the following:

- A Living Trust

- A Division of Assets

- A Durable Power of Attorney for Finances

- A Durable Power of Attorney for Health.

To cope psychologically:
- Stay informed about current findings relating to Alzheimer's disease

- Do not worry about the things you *cannot* do — concentrate on the things you *can* do

- Maintain your sense of humor

- Avoid stress.

To cope practically:

- Learn all you can about the way the disease is affecting you

- Establish a structured daily routine

- Maintain good physical and nutritional health.

To stay entertained:

- Maintain as many interests as you can for as long as you can

- Participate in outside activities

- Take advantage of this time to fulfill personal and family goals.

Yes, Alzheimer's disease has many negatives. That does not mean *you* have to be negative. You have a rare opportunity to redesign your life by stressing all the things that can make your life richer, despite Alzheimer's disease. When you think this way, you have that "open and positive" attitude that motivates you to act. You can then begin to enrich the quality of your life. ■

How Can I Put Meaning Back Into My Life?

This question is difficult to answer because people find meaning in different things. Our answer comes in two parts:

- Those things that gave your life meaning before you had Alzheimer's should continue to give it meaning now. Remember, your life had plenty of meaning before your diagnosis, so there were many months when your life had meaning while you had Alzheimer's disease, but didn't know it. This proves you can have a meaningful life with the disease. If meaning was not a problem before your diagnosis, it need not be a problem now. Continue to cultivate those things in your life that make it meaningful. Take the extra free time you now have to enhance that meaning even more.

- If you feel that Alzheimer's disease is robbing you of the things that make life meaningful, you may need to do some soul-searching. You have made a serious error if you derive meaning from anything that can be taken away from you, such as your job, the ability to drive a car, or even a relationship. The problem with basing meaning in your life on anything temporal is that when it is gone, so is your life's meaning.

If Alzheimer's disease has robbed you of that which gave your life meaning, we feel very deeply for you. We suggest that you try to find meaning that cannot be taken away. For some, that may come through trusting God. For others, it may be found by working on their own character. Find out what it is for you and deepen that part of your life.

Do not get stuck regretting endlessly what you do not have. Develop an independence of spirit that finds meaning in who you *can* be. ■

How Can I Gain More Respect From People?

With so many things going wrong, and with the frustration of not being able to do things that you did in the past, it is easy to lose your sense of self. You may feel that you are worthless and good for nothing. When you feel this way, it is hard for you to imagine how others can respect you. Consider the following:

You have done many worthwhile things in your life. Those who know you respect you for those things, and who you are. That you do not function at the same level now does not detract from what you have already accomplished.

How you deal with the changes of Alzheimer's disease will make a big difference in how people feel and react towards you. The better you deal with your illness, and the more you continue to stay involved with others, the more respect you will receive. ■

How Can I Fill My Free Time?

Finding creative and useful ways to fill your time is essential. Since most patients cannot hold a job, you may have difficulty finding constructive ways to fill your time.

Spend part of each day exercising and walking. Both are extremely beneficial to an Alzheimer's patient.

Reflect on your personal goals. What have you always said you would do, if only you had the time? Spend more time with your family? Travel? Donate time to a good cause? This is your chance to achieve those goals.

Should your goals not take you away from home, be sure to build regular outside activities into your schedule. Visit friends, attend concerts, or visit senior centers. Do something that gives you regular social interaction.

Still, there will be times when you are home alone with nothing to do. What then? TV and radio are obvious choices. Following is a list of other suggestions:

- Listen to records, tapes or CDs

- Play tapes of old radio shows or listen to books-on-tape

- Get a pet for company

- Read for as long as you can — enjoy the visual delight of art, photography books and your family pictures

- Arts-and-Crafts projects are difficult for many patients, but others can still enjoy them

- Jigsaw puzzles are fun for many, but can be frustrating for those with visual/spatial problems

- Write or record your autobiography, or the story of your family.

- Create a cookbook by compiling the recipes for dishes you have served your family, and pass it on to your children.

Please add your own ideas to this list, and ask your caregiver for more suggestions. The book *Failure Free Activities for the Alzheimer's Patient*, listed in Appendix B, has many excellent suggestions.

We realize that your participation in any activity may not be at the level that you participated in the past, but you can still enjoy being active on a different level. It is crucial that you not allow self-pity to prevent you from achieving your goals. *If you feel sorry for yourself, you will waste the rest of your life.*

Do not be negative. This is your chance to achieve your goals. You and your caregiver just need to find a method that works for you. If you stay open to creative alternatives, many of your goals can still be achieved. ■

How Can I Achieve My Goals?

You may need to adjust your expectations in order to achieve your goals. You need to be realistic about your abilities and limitations, and creative about how you achieve your goals. There comes a point when patients can best achieve their goals by working with a partner. Be willing to include a friend or your caregiver. Consider hiring someone to help, if you need to, but *do* try to achieve your goals. Here are two examples that show how a patient can make adjustments in order to achieve a goal:

Example One: The Trip

A couple wanted to tour Europe by car. However, the husband developed Alzheimer's disease and it became unsafe for him to drive. He adjusted his expectation; they joined an organized tour and saw Europe by coach. It was not the trip they planned, but it was still a fine trip.

Example Two: The Hobby

We know one man who is a nut for flowers. He wanted to become a tour leader at the Botanical Gardens after he retired. Then he was diagnosed with Alzheimer's disease. It affected him in such a way that he could not lecture. However, he adjusted his expectations and he still goes to the Botanical Gardens regularly. He is responsible for tending a particular section. This is within his abilities; it gives him an interest and responsibility outside the house; and he is doing something he loves. He was disappointed that he could not lecture, but he found a creative way of working at the Botanical Gardens anyway.

A good way to *never* achieve a goal is to get mad and swear that you will only do it *your* way, or not at all. If you can compromise and work within your limitations, you can achieve many of your goals. ∎

WHY CAN'T I REMEMBER
HOW TO DO SIMPLE THINGS?

Alzheimer's affects your memory because it affects your brain. Brains work when brain cells function properly, and individual cells work together. Alzheimer's disease slowly stops the communication between cells, so they cannot work together. It also kills individual cells. This eventually affects all the functions of the brain, but most Alzheimer's patients first notice the effects on their memory. When you have trouble with your memory, you will have difficulty doing simple things. ■

Should I Practice The Skills I Am Losing?

The decision to practice the skills you are losing depends on the potential danger of the activity and on how frustrated you feel when you practice.

If you are losing your driving skills or your ability to work a buzz saw or a gas oven, you should not practice. *Some activities are too dangerous.* If you are not at your best, you could injure yourself. If you have any questions about whether a skill is potentially dangerous, talk to your caregiver.

Other skills, like practicing your handwriting or reviewing things that you have forgotten, are not dangerous. Many patients find that practice helps reinforce these skills for a while. If you want to practice, and if practice helps, then do it.

There may be things you can do to compensate for a skill that you appear to be losing. Work with your family and health professionals to find out what is helpful. Be flexible, and keep a positive attitude.

When the time comes that practice leads only to frustration, it is time to stop practicing. Turn your attention to those things you can do for yourself. ∎

WILL I EVER GET BETTER?

Alzheimer's is a progressive disease. This means the disease will get worse, not better.

Like everyone else, you will have good and bad days. After a bad day, you may feel as if you have improved a bit. Enjoy it for as long as it lasts. Unfortunately, another bad day will eventually come.

Sometimes patients feel improvements in concentration due to experimental Alzheimer's medications. They may also feel more motivated. However, these improvements are not experienced by *all* patients. We hope that these drugs, once developed, will slow, prevent, or cure Alzheimer's disease. ∎

How Hard Should I Try To Do Things?

There is a difference between pushing yourself to the best of your ability and frustrating yourself by trying to do something that is no longer possible for you to do. Alzheimer's disease destroys brain cells and certain cells govern certain activities. They do not regenerate, so you will not be able to get those skills back.

You should stop trying when you become frustrated. Frustration is a sign that it is time to concentrate on the things you can do more easily. You gain nothing by pushing yourself to anger and frustration. ■

IF THIS DISEASE IS GOING TO WIN IN THE END, WHY BOTHER FIGHTING IT?

This question is very deceptive, because it seems logical. If the disease will win, you think that fighting it is futile. However, this way of thinking does not take into account the fact that there may be many years before you die. Let's ask the question in a new way, considering these years: *Do you want your remaining years to be good or bad?* When put this way the choice is obvious.

The disease may win in the end but, in the meantime, you want the best life you can have. Fighting Alzheimer's disease is your best chance of making those years *good* years. ■

Why Can't I Continue Doing The Activities I've Been Doing For Most Of My Life?

Many patients reason that since they have been doing something most of their lives, they should be allowed to continue. We hear this most often when patients are told to give up driving and handling their finances.

Remember that you have not had Alzheimer's most of your life, and Alzheimer's disease changes you. You may now remember how to fill out a check, how to record it, even how to pay bills with it. But Alzheimer's will make you forget. Patients have forgotten to pay bills, and even forgotten second and third notices. They wondered why their power and water were turned off. They wrote a check, but forgot to record the amount in their checkbook. They then wrote other checks for more money than they had in their account.

Someday, you will not be able to handle your finances without making mistakes, and you will not know about your mistakes until it is too late. When your caregiver asks you to give up your finances, do so. It may hurt your pride a little, but that is better than paying the consequences for serious financial mistakes.

The same is true for driving. Perhaps you did not get lost last time, but you *will* eventually. There are *no* exceptions. It does not matter how long you have been driving, or that you have never been lost, had an accident, or a ticket. If you continue driving, all these things *will* happen. The only question is *when*.

You must stop driving and handling your finances so that you can *prevent* traffic accidents and financial errors from happening. You will be happier if you can accept these limitations, rather than resisting them. ■

WILL I KNOW IF I MAKE MISTAKES?

Sometimes you *will* know that you have made a mistake, but occasionally you will *not*. For example, you will know if you cannot think of a word you want; you may not notice a mathematical error, however.

The problem is that some mistakes are more serious than others. Picking the wrong word is not very serious, but some Alzheimer's patients have gone into bankruptcy by making mistakes with their finances. Others have started fires by forgetting they put dinner on to cook. There is no question that Alzheimer's disease has limited your abilities.

The rule of thumb is: If there is something you can safely do, do it. If you can only do a part, do that. For example, you may want to cook and you remember how. The danger is that you might forget the food is in the oven. In this case, you can help prepare the food, but be sure someone else is there to keep an eye on it.

This will allow you to be as active and useful as you can. It is important for you to acknowledge your need for help and to put your trust in others. If you cannot do this, you will bring on much hardship with your more serious mistakes. ■

What If My Mistakes
Have Serious Consequences?

Your mistakes can have *very* serious consequences. Many Alzheimer's patients have insisted on living their lives as if they were not ill. As a result, they have put themselves into bankruptcy, started fires, and been lost for days.

Remember the saying: *an ounce of prevention is worth a pound of cure.* You can help to prevent mistakes by taking the disease seriously. Alzheimer's is changing you in such a way that you can no longer do as much as you *believe* you can. You need to rely on the advice of your caregiver for what you should continue to do and what you must trust to others. Caregivers see mistakes that the disease prevents you from noticing. Listen to them and accept their help. That is the ounce of prevention that can save you from needing the pound of cure.

There is one other thing you can do. Let's say you've made a bad mistake and now have to pay serious consequences. Let that experience teach you to prevent mistakes in the future. Learn that the time has come to get serious about your new limitations. Use this as an opportunity to *not make that mistake again.* Make these changes while you can still decide to act:

- Get a Living Will
- Get a Living Trust
- Get a Durable Power of Attorney for finances
- Get a Durable Power of Attorney for health
- Do not drive
- Do not cook when you are alone
- Have someone check your finances.

By acknowledging that you have Alzheimer's disease and adjusting your life accordingly, you may prevent those mistakes that carry the biggest consequences. ■

Why Have A Sense Of Humor?
There Is Nothing Funny About Alzheimer's.

Having a neurological disease is not funny. Neither is war or crime. People are complex. We tend to find something to laugh about, no matter how bad life gets. It may be the behavior of a pet, a comedy show, or a silly mistake, but laughter asserts itself into our lives. It is inevitable. Alzheimer's may not be funny, but life is.

There are many reasons to have a sense of humor. Humor relieves stress. It gives delight. It makes you feel closer to others. Humor expresses feelings and relaxes the atmosphere. It helps keep things in perspective.

Laughter may not be the *best* medicine, but it *is* very therapeutic. ■

How Can I Keep My Sense Of Humor?

Having Alzheimer's disease can be very stressful, and stress is bad for you. Relieving stress is important. Humor is our natural and wonderful stress-reliever.

Except during periods of depression, maintaining your sense of humor is surprisingly easy. Just live your life, and you will find reasons to laugh.

Very little seems funny during a depression. See your doctor or counselor to cope with the clinical problems of depression. Try not to get angry or upset with your mistakes; laugh at them instead. See the humor in life and in yourself. If you can, it will make life much more pleasant for you, your family, and your friends. ■

IF I AM GOING TO DIE ANYWAY, WHY SHOULD I STAY HEALTHY?

Staying healthy will give you the best possible quality of life in the time you have left. By staying healthy you can prolong much of your independence, possibly by a few years. By letting yourself go, you risk prolonging the time spent depending on others, including time spent in a nursing home. Most patients want to be independent for as long as possible. The best way to do this is through good physical health. ■

What Should I Do
When I Feel Confused Or Afraid?

When you feel confused or afraid, there is something you must *not* do. Do not panic. *To panic is to lose control.*

The more stress you have, the harder it will be to remember things you normally know. Your fear and confusion are just momentary.

To regain control of yourself and the situation, sit down, take some deep breaths, and give yourself a chance to think. Look around slowly, and try to pick up any signs or cues that will help end your confusion. If someone you know is nearby, tell them how you feel. Sometimes just telling someone you trust that you feel frightened helps dispel the fear. ■

How Should I Handle My Anger?

Let's look at the three kinds of anger Alzheimer's patients typically have:

- ANGER AT HAVING THE DISEASE. When something bad happens, people often react with anger. It may be a divorce, the loss of a job, or a death in the family. We get mad. That is perfectly normal, even inevitable. The trick is not to become so consumed by the anger that you cannot function in the rest of your life.

  The healthy way to handle this anger is to admit that you have it, and acknowledge that your anger is okay. You will only prolong its effects by denying it.

  Be willing to talk about it to family and friends. Tell them how you feel and why. If it would help, see a professional counselor. When you do not need to feel the anger anymore, it will pass. Talking about it is part of the process that helps it pass.

- ANGER STEMMING FROM FRUSTRATION. An Alzheimer's patient has a lot to feel frustrated about. You feel frustrated whenever you cannot do something you used to do. You feel frustrated when others try to do too much for you. It is frustrating to be constantly corrected. You have more going on in your mind than others give you credit for, so you feel frustrated. Frustration leads to anger at whatever is frustrating you.

  The solution is the same. Talk it out. Tell your friends, family or a counselor how you feel and why. Articulate it as best you can until they understand. You may also want to talk to the person who frustrates you. Tell them you are frustrated by the way they help you when you do not need help, or by the way they constantly correct you. Tell them how you want to be treated in the future. Specify how you want them to behave when you need help, as well as when you do not need help.

You may have trouble organizing all those ideas and conversations. Take your time. If it would help, write it down or speak into a tape recorder to play later. You can show them this page as a place to begin the conversation. Do not let them continue to frustrate you.

- **ANGER FOR NO IDENTIFIABLE REASON.** The disease can cause flashes of rage where a patient will lash out in anger, usually at those who are closest to them. These incidents pass as quickly as they come, and the patient seldom remembers them. When they occur, they are unfortunate; but they are part of the disease. It is a phase that will eventually pass. If anger becomes a problem, see your doctor. There are medications that can help. ■

What Can I Do About My Depression?

By recognizing that you are depressed and asking this question, you have already taken the first step in doing something about it. Depression can be treated. Depression does not only make you feel sad, it can make your memory problems worse.

There are two general types of depression. The first is called "reactive" depression. With reactive depression, patients are depressed because they have memory problems. This type of depression can be helped by joining a support group, talking to a psychiatrist or counselor, and by participating in stimulating outside activities. A combination of the three can help even more.

The second type, called "Major Depressive Disorder" is due to a chemical imbalance. The symptoms are usually more severe than with reactive depression. It should be treated by a psychiatrist and the use of anti-depressant medication. Treatment with anti-depressants requires a four-to-six week trial so that the medication can build up in your body. You will not feel results until the medication reaches a certain level. As well as taking medication, engage in outside activities and a regular exercise program. These combined steps may help you recover from depression faster.

Asking this question was just the first step. Now take the next step. Talk to your doctor about which treatment is best for you. ■

DO I HAVE TO TALK ABOUT MY FEELINGS?

No, you do not *have* to talk about your feelings. The reason we urge you to is that we want you to cope with the emotional difficulties caused by Alzheimer's disease in the best way you can. Talking about your feelings is a tool for doing this. When you refuse to discuss your feelings, you deny yourself the use of a very helpful tool. It makes sense to use every tool at your disposal to deal with this disease. ∎

CAN PSYCHOLOGICAL COUNSELING HELP ME AND MY FAMILY?

Yes, psychological counseling can help. The earlier you see a counselor, the more help you can receive. It is very traumatic for patients to learn that they have Alzheimer's disease. The diagnosis and their awareness of their mental decline leaves them anxious, depressed and frustrated. They are under much stress.

New research suggests that prolonged stress may accelerate the progress of Alzheimer's disease. Early counseling can help reduce stress and depression, improve self-esteem, and help you maintain your sense of dignity. It may even slow the progress of the disease and help patients function more effectively.

Counseling can help family members as well. They too experience anger, depression, and frustration. They also bear an increasing responsibility to take care of you and your household. We recommend counseling to ease this burden. Counseling may be individual, with couples, or as a family. It can be with a single counselor or a support group. These things are determined by your needs. Your doctor or another health care professional can help you find the counseling situation that works for you. Many health care plans provide coverage for this kind of counseling.

Counseling makes sense. If you believe that a family member needs counseling, urge them to seek help, and consider it for yourself. ■

Why Should I Join A Support Group?

Here are four reasons to join a support group:

- To benefit from the experiences of others. You are not the first person to have the disease. Alzheimer's creates many problems in your daily life. You and your caregiver can talk about specific problems at a support group and get suggestions from those who have already faced your problem.

- It gives you the opportunity to talk. It is therapeutic to talk to sympathetic people about the frustrations caused by Alzheimer's disease. Simply getting to know other people with the same problem is a comfort to many.

- A support group is a safe forum to bring up issues that might be hard to talk about at home. For example, let's pretend you are frustrated because your caregiver corrects you. You want her to stop, but, for some reason, you can't talk to her directly. You or your caregiver can raise this problem in a support group, where the objectivity of others can help your caregiver think about the issue.

- A support group is an excellent way to learn about Alzheimer's research, community resources, and the legal issues facing you. Other members of the group will know many things you want to learn.

As the disease progresses, you may not be able to participate as actively in the support group, but you can still enjoy the company. It is also a place to meet new friends and expand your social life. ■

It Would Help To Talk To Other Alzheimer's Patients. How Can I Find Them?

To meet other people affected by Alzheimer's disease, contact your local chapter of the Alzheimer's Association and ask them the time and location of the closest Alzheimer's support group. Patients and caregivers there are an excellent source of ideas, information and advice. It is wonderful that you want to take this step. This is an important way to cope with the practical and emotional frustrations of having Alzheimer's disease. ■

Why Isn't My Doctor Doing More For Me?

There are things your doctor can do, but there are also things your doctor *cannot* do. Your doctor cannot cure Alzheimer's disease or slow down its effects. Your doctor can do these six things.

- Your doctor can make a diagnosis, which in your case has probably already been done.

- Your doctor can monitor the progress of Alzheimer's disease in you, and keep you informed of those areas where you can expect the most difficulty.

- Your doctor can continue to treat you for medical problems not related to Alzheimer's disease.

- Your doctor can treat you for *some* medical problems caused by Alzheimer's disease. Incontinence and sleeplessness can sometimes be treated; loss of memory cannot.

- Your doctor can give practical advice to you and your family on how to compensate for some of the mental abilities you lose through Alzheimer's disease.

- Your doctor can keep you abreast of the latest findings and treatments.

Some doctors have more experience with Alzheimer's disease than others. The more experience, the better informed their judgment and advice will be. If your doctor has little experience with Alzheimer's disease and you want someone with more, you have the right to change doctors. Remember, there are no miracles out there. All doctors are limited in what they can do for you. ■

Should I Change To A Different Doctor?

When patients ask this question, they generally want to know one of two things:

- Is there another doctor who could prescribe a treatment or medication that will reverse or cure Alzheimer's disease? The answer to that is no.

- Is there a doctor who can do more for me than my doctor can? Possibly.

Ask yourself these questions:

- IS YOUR DOCTOR INTERESTED IN WORKING WITH OLDER PATIENTS? Your doctor should be knowledgeable about working with older patients who have dementia or Alzheimer's disease.

- IS YOUR DOCTOR KNOWLEDGEABLE ABOUT ALZHEIMER'S DISEASE? Patients have many practical problems. Experienced physicians can help you find solutions. They are aware of the physical ailments that sometimes follow Alzheimer's disease, and can treat those problems.

- DO YOU AND YOUR FAMILY FEEL COMFORTABLE TALKING TO YOUR PHYSICIAN? Some of your problems may be embarrassing. You need a doctor with whom you can be completely honest.

- IS YOUR DOCTOR AVAILABLE WHEN NEEDED? Alzheimer's related problems can arise frequently. It is important to have a doctor you can reach when needed.

If the answer to these questions is yes, then you would do well to stay with your present physician. Your doctor is qualified to treat Alzheimer's disease, and already knows you and your family.

If you feel that your present doctor does not meet the criteria, you may want to consider a change. If you decide to change, you can find another physician by contacting your local Alzheimer's Association for a list of doctors in your area who specialize in Geriatrics or Gero-psychiatry. You may also consult your local County Medical Society, and members of an Alzheimer's support group. ■

My Doctor Did Not Really Explain What I Have, And Does Not Care!

It is possible that you have an uncaring doctor, but there is probably another explanation. Studies which were conducted to learn how patients take the bad news of a diagnosis showed that patients hear little more than the diagnosis itself. One of the writers of this book had a relative with Alzheimer's disease. The patient first spent a half-hour with his wife and doctor; then the rest of the family joined them for 45 minutes. The doctor explained the disease, discussed what we could expect in the future, and answered questions, all in a very sensitive but professional manner. He ended by giving us an information package to read at our leisure. Weeks later, this relative claimed we had only a brief meeting, where the doctor gave the bad news and then went home. He said his doctor did not care.

Most patients remember hearing their diagnosis this way, no matter what actually happened. If your doctor is insensitive, you should find another doctor. However, you should not use the time of your diagnosis to measure your doctor's interest; it is better to judge the doctor's subsequent dealings with you. Talk it over with your family. If they agree that your doctor is insensitive to you, it may be appropriate to find another physician. ■

Will Alzheimer's Disease
Cause My Body To Change?

Your body will not change very much in the early stages of the disease. There will be eventual changes, but these will not develop until quite late. Patients then tend to stoop and develop a shuffle in their walks, because many develop Parkinson's-like changes in the central nervous system. This causes stiffening, leading to slower movements.

Alzheimer's disease can also affect the way many patients perceive depth and distance, and how they see complicated patterns. A black tile on a white floor can appear three-dimensional and you may try to step over it, so this can affect the way you walk.

Stooping and shuffling may be postponed by regular exercise and walking exercise. These exercises should enable you to walk for longer than you otherwise would. Reports state that patients who have already begun to change often improve when they begin to walk and exercise regularly.

Myoclonic Movements affect some patients. These are usually an involuntary movement of the arms or legs, an unexpected jerk or twitch.

Many patients also lose their sense of smell. This is not harmful, but has the unfortunate effect of making meals seem bland.

Some patients lose weight, despite eating healthy amounts of good food. This only occurs in the late stages of Alzheimer's, and the reason for it is unknown. Weight loss may have a cause unrelated to Alzheimer's disease. Please consult a doctor if you undergo an unexpected loss in weight. ■

WHAT SHOULD I DO
IF I AM HAVING A BAD DAY?

An Alzheimer's patient often knows if they are having a bad day before they even get out of bed. After waking, they will feel more vague than usual.

A technique that can help turn a bad day into a good one is to take your time before getting up. Laze in bed for a while. Have a glass of orange juice before rising. Let your caregiver know that you are having a bad day and need to take things slowly.

Taking this time helps many patients get a better grip on the day. ■

WILL I WAKE UP ONE MORNING
AND NOT BE ABLE TO DO ANYTHING?

No, there are usually no dramatic overnight changes with Alzheimer's disease.

Everybody has good days and bad days. You are no exception. There will be some days when you will seem to have lost many of your mental abilities overnight. Don't panic. You are just having a bad day. A day or two later, you may find yourself functioning quite well, almost like before you had Alzheimer's. That is just the ebb and flow of good and bad days that all of us have. They are just more noticeable when you have Alzheimer's.

Here is a list of some of the things that can create a bad day:

- Illness

- The unkindness of others

- Stress

- Fear

- Being away from home

- Bewildering surroundings, (such as being in a crowd).

Sickness and *confusion* are also problems. When Alzheimer's patients become physically ill, it can affect them profoundly. It may leave them feeling like someone who has had Alzheimer's for a very long time. As the illness passes, they can expect their mental faculties to return to the way they were before they became sick.

Because Alzheimer's patients have trouble taking in and understanding what is going on around them, they sometimes find themselves in unfamiliar and frightening situations that cause them to panic. They draw a blank and do not know how to respond. This is a temporary problem. When they get away from whatever is frightening or confusing them, they can become their usual selves again. ■

WILL I KNOW IF I MAKE BAD DECISIONS?

Making good decisions will become difficult. Decision-making depends on three things:

- Your knowledge of facts and ideas

- Your ability to remember past experiences

- Your ability to analyze facts, ideas and experience to make a new decision.

Alzheimer's disease blocks access to your knowledge and memories and impedes your ability to process information. This is why your decisions may not be as wise as they once were. Alzheimer's is so tricky that you may not realize it has impaired your judgment. Patients need people they can trust to help them make decisions.

Be open with your family and friends. If you let them know you have a problem remembering, they can assist you as you think through a decision, and suggest possible alternatives that you might not see.

Some patients have trouble trusting. They end up hurting themselves in the long run, because they will not accept help when they need it. It is important for you to believe that Alzheimer's disease has changed your life, and you now need help making decisions. There is now a greater risk of making a bad decision than of someone betraying you.

Learning to trust is essential. ■

WHY DO PEOPLE KEEP TELLING ME WHAT TO DO?

Frustrating, isn't it? You are about to do something, like change your clothes or set the table. You pause for a moment to remember the next step. Just as you figure it out, someone tells you what to do.

If you are like most patients, you feel a bit angry at such times. You knew what to do. You figured it out. You did not need help, and now you do not feel you are being treated with the respect you deserve. You are probably right. But let's look at the other point of view.

Alzheimer's disease slows down your reactions. The person who told you what to do sees you pause. They thought you were not sure what to do next. They were right. For a moment, you did not. As they tried to help, you figured it out by yourself. You did not need their help *this* time, but there *will* be times when you do.

You need to communicate. Talk to them, write a note, make a tape-recording, or ask them to read this page. Do whatever you need to do to help them understand that your mind is keener than they think. Ask them to give you more time before they tell you what to do. The time required will get longer as the disease progresses. Make them understand that.

On the other hand, they are only trying to help. They are not trying to insult you. If you want to be fair, try to remember that.

One solution is to work out a cue with the people you know. Suggest that they do not help until you ask for it, either verbally or by using an agreed-upon hand gesture. By keeping the lines of communication open, you should be able to work out a way of getting help when you need it, while having unwanted help pushed on you less often. As always, communication is very important. ■

WHY DOES MY CAREGIVER SAY "NO"?

Since Alzheimer's is a disease affecting memory, forgetfulness becomes a problem. You may think you remember how to do something, but you get it wrong. You may want to do the right thing at the wrong time. You may have just finished doing something, forgotten you did it, and want to do it again. To keep you from making these mistakes, your caregiver tells you no.

That is fine, as far as it goes. You do not want to make mistakes. The problem is that constantly hearing no can make you feel bad about yourself and frustrated with your caregiver. If this is a problem for you, have your caregiver read this page, or find some way to give them this message yourself.

There is usually an alternative to using the word no. Here are some suggestions you can share with your caregiver:

- In a case where you do not remember how to do something, and so try to do it the wrong way, your caregiver can say, "That might work better if you did it like this," instead of, "No, that's not how to do it."

- Should you try to do the right thing at the wrong time, your caregiver can say, "Let's do that later," rather than, "No, it isn't time yet."

- If you begin a task you've already completed, a simple, "Honey, maybe you forgot, but you already took care of that," is much better than, "No, you already did that."

Caregivers *often* jump the gun in saying no or in giving advice. Alzheimer's disease slows your response time, so it takes a bit longer to assimilate information. A caregiver who waits for you to "get it" helps more than a caregiver who responds with a quick yes or no.

It is tough enough to live with Alzheimer's disease without also experiencing the verbal battering of constantly hearing no. Find a way to help your caregiver stop correcting you in this negative way, and to begin helping you positively. ■

WHY DOES MY CAREGIVER YELL AT ME?

Think back to the years before you were diagnosed with Alzheimer's disease. Didn't your caregiver sometimes yell at you then? Of course they did. People sometimes yell, and the reason is usually frustration.

Your caregiver's frustration can be caused by any number of things that have nothing to do with you, though the yelling is directed at you. That is not fair, but it happens to everyone. Try to accept it and not take it personally.

As your disease grows worse and you make more mistakes, or are slower to react, your caregiver's frustration may grow as well. Chances are your caregiver will still take it out on you sometimes, but their frustration is really with their inability to help you. In fact, most caregivers get upset with themselves when they yell at you. You will feel better when you talk about it.

If this becomes a real problem, suggest that you both get counseling. A counselor can teach your caregiver techniques to cope with frustration and can help you gain a better under-standing of the problem. ■

How Can I Overcome My Loneliness?

Everyone needs to feel connected to someone who cares for them and can be relied upon in times of need. Yet people with memory problems often narrow their contacts with friends and family as a way of avoiding embarrassment.

It does not work. It isolates patients and makes friends and family uncomfortable. People who are uncomfortable with you tend to stay away from you.

Acknowledge that you contribute to your loneliness by being self-protective. Then, reach out to others and be open about your problem. You must try to stop feeling embarrassed; discuss your memory problems with your family and friends.

Once that is behind you, there are further steps you can take to overcome loneliness. You should be willing to:

- Try new things

- Join a support group

- Join an activity program.

Taking the initiative to do these things may be frightening. If you have family, ask them to help. If you are alone, ask your doctor to suggest an agency that can assist you.

Having memory loss is a chronic illness, like heart disease or diabetes. You are not crazy or inept, and you have not failed to try hard enough. There is no need to feel embarrassed. You have years ahead of you when you can still do and enjoy many things, including the company of others. Make the most of this opportunity, and overcome your loneliness by reaching out to others. ■

It Is So *Hard* To Socialize; Should I Continue?

Socializing becomes increasingly challenging as a result of the disease process; all Alzheimer's patients struggle with this. It is difficult to keep up with others in conversation, and it is hard to get in your contribution before everyone moves on.

Even though it is frustrating, it is important to maintain social contacts. You share a basic human need for the company of others. If you stop interacting with others, you will become depressed and experience increased problems with your memory. *You must not stop interacting with others.*
Here are some tricks you can use to make socializing more enjoyable:

- AVOID SITUATIONS THAT MAKE YOU FEEL UNCOMFORTABLE. For most patients, these are unstructured and noisy gatherings, like cocktail parties or noisy restaurants.

- ADJUST YOUR EXPECTATIONS. Accept that you have slowed down. Enjoy yourself on the level you can by listening to interesting people or watching the fun. If you want to actively participate, do not be embarrassed to raise a hand for attention and have everybody wait for you. Take your time. If someone does not let you finish, tell them you have not yet finished, and continue.

- INVITE FRIENDS TO THE KIND OF SOCIAL ACTIVITY MOST COMFORTABLE FOR YOU. Go to a concert or a movie. Invite them for a hike in an interesting neighborhood or park. Have them over for a barbecue or picnic.

Although you have trouble expressing yourself, there are still many ways for you to enjoy group activities. It just requires some adjustments and a little extra planning. ■

How Can I Get People To Let Me Participate In A Conversation?

You need to find a way to participate in conversations that works for you. We can make a number of suggestions, but the solution must be practical, and you must feel comfortable doing it. Following are two suggestions.

- **Let people know that you plan to participate in the conversation.** There are many ways to do this. You can tell them. You can put up a banner announcing it. Or you could get someone to help you make a card to give to your listeners. However you tell them, you must make it clear that you may be slow having your say, and that they should be patient and not interrupt until you have finished.

- **Use a signal to let people know when you want to take your turn.** Find a signal that works for you, and then explain that you will be using it. Hold up a hand for attention and when you get it, start speaking. Keep your hand up until you finish, so others will know not to interrupt.

This may sound a little extreme, but a red ping-pong paddle would be a great attention-getter. Raise it when you want to speak and wait for everyone to listen. Then keep it up as a signal that you have more to say, even if you pause. Do not lower the paddle until you have made your contribution.

We realize you may not feel comfortable bringing a ping-pong paddle to a dinner party. However, the goal is to get you and your caregiver to find a way to get and keep the attention of others while you have your rightful say. A speech therapist can suggest excellent strategies to manage these problems. Good luck! ■

What Should I Do If I Cannot Find The Words To Say What I Mean?

Not being able to find the words to say what you mean is very frustrating for an Alzheimer's patient. We sympathize if this happens to you. Try to remember that you are the one putting pressure on yourself to find the word. One of the things that blocks your memory is that pressure. The best way to find the word is to relax. We know that is easier said than done. Here are five things you can do:

- Take your time. Let a few minutes pass if you need to. Think through what you want to say and try again.

- Find another word that means the same thing, or start your sentence over with a fresh approach.

- Go to another room and speak into a tape recorder. You have taken a break and a change of scenery by leaving the room. The tape will let you record your idea while you are alone, so you need not feel the pressure of a conversation.

- Write down your idea; then read it to your listener, or show it to them. Making that transition from speaking to writing may give you the words you need.

- Have your caregiver there, ready to help. Work out a cue, like nodding or pointing your finger when you want your caregiver to suggest a word or to complete your sentence.

Some patients have cue cards with a picture on one side and the word printed on the other. Do whatever you need to do to make the best of your situation. Do not be embarrassed. Admit your problem, and you will find that your listeners will usually bear with you. ■

CAN A SPEECH THERAPIST HELP ME?

Speech therapists have begun to take an active interest in Alzheimer's patients. They have developed many ingenious ways for patients to communicate when words fail them. They find out where you need the most help and develop an individualized program geared to your needs. If you would like help, ask your health care professional or the Alzheimer's Association to recommend a therapist to you. ■

I Took Care Of Everyone Else, Why Can't They Take Care Of Me Now?

We understand the anger that makes you say that. You've given a lot to others and deserve to get something back. It may help if you consider these three things:

- Alzheimer's disease will increase the amount of care you need. The longer you have this disease, the more care you require. No matter how much your family loves you, there will come a point where they can no longer care for you alone.

- Caring for an Alzheimer's patient is stressful for the caregiver, more stressful than caring for a child. Caregivers have a higher rate of physical illness than others. They need a balanced life outside caregiving to maintain their mental and physical well-being. Should your caregiver get sick, you would have to go to a nursing home anyway. The best time to go is when your caregiver is healthy and can find the right place for you.

- Going to a nursing home does not mean your caregiver will no longer care for you. They can still care for you in a nursing home, where the environment is better structured, and you will receive the additional care you need.

- Be fair to your caregiver. You may need to go to a nursing home, but they have been taking good care of you for a long time. Try not to let your feelings blind you to all they have done in the past. ∎

CAN I AVOID BECOMING A BURDEN TO MY CHILDREN?

There is a difference between needing help and becoming a burden. You will need help in a number of ways as your disease progresses.

You will need help managing your financial affairs, in coping with the activities of daily living, and with transportation, to name but three. How you choose to handle this issue will make a difference in whether or not you become a burden to others.

You must acknowledge the situation and work with others to plan for your needs, rather than insist there is nothing wrong. *Accepting help* is the key to whether others feel burdened. The burden comes when you need help, but refuse to accept it. That burdens others because they now have to try to help you in spite of yourself.

We know it is frightening and difficult to accept that you cannot manage alone. However, accepting your need is the difference between receiving help and putting a burden on others. ■

Who Will Help Me If I Am Alone?

You do not have to feel alone; you have many options.

First, you must accept that you will need help. When you accept that, you can explore your options and select the kind of help you want.

Start with your family. Even if they do not live nearby, there is probably someone willing to oversee your affairs from a distance. They can work with a local agency to provide day-to-day assistance.

Do you have friends? Choose one who is trustworthy and capable to oversee your affairs and provide emotional support.

If you can afford it, you can have live-in help. This ought to be handled through an agency, to provide outside supervision. It can be costly and disorienting to a patient in the later stages of Alzheimer's disease. Plan early to take best advantage of this option.

If you cannot afford full-time help, there are a number of agencies that can help you with shopping, transportation and assist with your finances. They can also arrange for someone to visit you regularly. There is a cost for this, but it is much less than for full-time help.

Also, plan early if you are going into a facility that offers full-time care. The daily cost is high, but most patients eventually need this extra care.

Your doctor, local agencies, social services and groups like Catholic Charities and the Agency on Aging are sources of information and help. Please contact them for further information. With all these alternatives, there is no reason to feel hopeless or even alone. Accept that you need help, and take an active role in deciding who will help. ■

Why Have Our Friends Abandoned Us?

When someone is diagnosed with Alzheimer's disease, they often find that some of their friends disappear. Many people are not strong enough to deal with the fact that someone they care about is sick. They are not rejecting you. They are coping with your disease the only way they can. They are frightened. They know if it can happen to you, then it can happen to them. It is a weakness on their part.

Try not to give in to feeling sorry for yourself. Some friends may have abandoned you, but think about the others who have not. Remember those who have remained faithful and what they mean to you.

If you are feeling alone, attend an Alzheimer's support group. Participants there know what you are going through. We have seen many important friendships develop at Alzheimer's support groups. ■

Do People Laugh At My Expense?

People are usually sympathetic to what you are experiencing. It is rare for someone to make fun of the problems that occur as a result of Alzheimer's disease.

Some patients occasionally feel that others are laughing at them. This happens when a joke is made in conversation, but the patient does not hear it fully. The laughter is mistaken for a joke at their expense. One way to overcome this feeling is to tell the person you did not hear the joke, and ask them to repeat it. You will usually find it had nothing to do with you. ■

WHAT IS DAYCARE?

Daycare is a social setting where you can spend time, and engage in structured activities. The term "daycare" is unfortunate because it invokes thoughts of babysitting for adults. For some people, it *is* that, but not for many others. A wide variety of people attend adult daycare, including many folks with a high degree of independence.

Daycare centers vary in terms of what they offer. You can expect most to serve meals and provide exercise classes as well as craft projects and music. Many have a library and a room in which you can socialize with other participants. As with everything in life, it is as good as *you* make it. Give yourself a chance to find a daycare center that can make your day stimulating and enjoyable. ■

WHY SHOULD I GO TO DAYCARE?

One of the best ways to take care of yourself is to keep your body and mind stimulated with exercise, conversation, and activities. It is wonderful to enjoy the company of your family, but you also need stimulation from outside your home.

Adult daycare gets you out of the house to a place where you can get the kind of physical and mental stimulation you need so much. Patients who do not participate in adult daycare usually do not fare as well as patients who do. It is in your best interest to attend.

Another issue is that caregivers need time off to run errands and have a life outside caregiving. The time you spend in adult daycare is time they can use to tend to other things. In this way, adult daycare is of benefit to both of you.

Many patients are apprehensive about adult daycare, but it offers many possibilities. You can choose the activities in which you participate, and those you want to skip. You can even choose which days you attend. Do not be put off because you tried it and did not like it. Other days will have different activities, and some centers are better than others. Try more than one, but please do try it. The stimulation it gives you can be of great benefit as you struggle with Alzheimer's disease. ■

WILL WE GO BROKE?

It can be very expensive to have Alzheimer's disease. The expense comes from two sources:

- NURSING CARE. This can mean anything from days spent in a daycare program, to nursing care in your home, to staying in a nursing home. All this costs money and those costs are rising. You and your caregiver should contact an attorney who specializes in elder law as soon as possible. They know the laws of your state and can help you position yourself to receive maximum state and federal benefits. Do not put this off, since some states require you to have everything in place long before you can receive maximum financial aid.

- PATIENTS WHO HANDLE THEIR OWN FINANCES CAN MAKE SERIOUS FINANCIAL MISTAKES. Since Alzheimer's disease causes memory problems, mistakes are made. Some patients have even gone bankrupt making serious financial errors. To guard against this, you need to have your caregiver double-check your finances to make sure the bills are paid, the work is done correctly, and the financial decisions are sound. You will eventually need to trust them with your finances.

Now we can answer the question, "Will you go broke?" It depends on how much you have, how well you position yourself legally, and on whether mistakes make you squander your financial resources. Please act quickly to protect yourself. ■

WHY SHOULD I SIGN
A DURABLE POWER OF ATTORNEY?

A durable power of attorney is a legal document in which you name the person who will handle your legal and financial affairs when you cannot do so yourself. You continue to handle your own affairs for as long as you are able; then the person you designate takes over without lengthy or costly legal maneuvers.

Many Alzheimer's patients do not want to sign a durable power of attorney. They fear losing control of their lives. However, it is really Alzheimer's disease that threatens their control, not the durable power of attorney.

Without a durable power of attorney, someone else will still handle your legal and financial business, but it may not be the person you choose. Your tool for controlling that choice is the durable power of attorney. ■

WHAT CAN I DO IF I FEEL I AM BEING PHYSICALLY OR EMOTIONALLY ABUSED?

If you feel you are being abused, talk about it with your doctor or social worker on your next visit. Contact them sooner, if you are still able, or have a friend contact them as well as Adult Protective Services.

Health and social workers can help you solve the problem. Help can range from finding out what is causing the problem and how to solve it, to finding a safer place for you to live.

It is imperative to talk to someone. Do not continue to suffer this abuse. ■

WHAT CAN I DO IF SOMEONE TAKES FINANCIAL ADVANTAGE OF ME?

Though rare, this *has* happened and is particularly difficult for an Alzheimer's patient to defend against. You cannot deal with it yourself, so get help. A trusted friend or family member is best. They can contact Adult Protective Services, the police, or an attorney. If you already have an attorney, and there is no one else you can trust, try to contact your lawyer directly.

If Alzheimer's has affected your ability to speak or dial the phone, help will be harder to find. Do your best to explain the problem verbally or in writing. It may be enough to show someone this page, and tell them the name of the person you believe is stealing from you.

Try to remember this: It is rare for anyone to take financial advantage of an Alzheimer's patient. It is more common for a patient to misunderstand someone's behavior and accuse them of stealing. Do your best not to make this mistake. ∎

Can The State Take All My Money?

No, the law will not permit the state to take all your money. It is not the state's money; it is *your* money. The only conceivable exception is if the state has to pay for your care.

If you are unable to care for yourself, and there is no one to care for you, and if you are the only one with legal access to your money or property, then the state can place a lien against your assets to help pay for your care. Only then can they touch what is yours, and they must spend it on you.

The law differs slightly from state to state. Consult a lawyer to get the information that applies to you. ∎

Can The State Put Me Away?

By law, the state can only put someone away if they are a danger to themselves or to others. Alzheimer's patients are seldom a danger to anyone. The only exception is when you cannot care for yourself, and nobody offers to care for you. Then a court assumes responsibility and places you where you can receive care. ∎

WILL MY SPOUSE GET TIRED OF TAKING CARE OF ME AND PUT ME AWAY?

We include the above question because patients do ask it, but the question misses the point. It makes two false assumptions:

- One false assumption is that you will be "put away." What an awful image that involves! To go into a nursing home is not to be "put away." You can leave for excursions with friends and family, and you can have visitors in to see you. It is a change, but it is not the end of everything.

- If you go to a nursing home, or other care facility, it will probably not be because your spouse is tired of taking care of you. It will be because you need more care than a non-professional can give. Moving to a nursing home does not mean you have been abandoned. It means your spouse needs help caring for you. Patients recognize the stress in their spouses, and begin to feel highly stressed themselves. They do better with specialized care.

Many patients are afraid that their spouses or caregivers will tire of taking care of them. Our experience has shown just the opposite. Caregivers often attempt to care for their spouses single-handedly, which is often way beyond their physical capabilities.

One of the best ways to help yourself is to have a positive attitude about yourself and your life. By seeing your spouse's role as caregiver and specialized care in an accurate light, you do yourself much good. It fosters the positive attitude that can help you so much.

Discuss this with your family soon. That will allow all of you to prepare for the kind of care you want to have. ■

WILL I HAVE TO GO TO A NURSING HOME?

You may have to go to a nursing home eventually, but you can delay the process. Throughout this book, we have suggested things you can do to keep your mind and body as sharp as possible. If you do these things, you may push back and shorten the time you will spend in a nursing home. Those things you can do are:

- Maintain a positive mental attitude

- Eat nutritious meals

- Exercise regularly

- Go on walks

- Stimulate the mind by seeing friends and going to cultural activities.

By keeping both mind and body as nimble as possible, you could delay going to a nursing home by many months, possibly by a few years.

We should also add that while most patients eventually need nursing care, some can avoid a nursing home with full-time live-in help. All nursing care is expensive, and live-in care is especially so. Prepare early for the financial burden that nursing care will bring your way. ■

Will I Reach A Point Where I Am No Longer Able To Communicate?

It is possible that at some point, you will no longer be able to communicate. Should Alzheimer's disease run its full course, it will steal your ability to communicate. However this is a late stage of the disease. It typically takes many years before this happens. ■

WILL I EVENTUALLY FORGET EVERYTHING?

No one can say with certainty that you will forget everything, since no one can probe the mind of another. The only honest answer is that if Alzheimer's disease runs its course, based on our current knowledge, we believe that you will. This comes only at the very end stage of the disease. ∎

WHY IS THERE A STIGMA ASSOCIATED WITH ALZHEIMER'S DISEASE?

Many diseases have a stigma. You are not being singled out. The stigma comes mostly from fear and helplessness. People are afraid of Alzheimer's disease because they do not want to get it themselves. They also want to help you, but feel helpless to do so. That makes them uncomfortable.

The best way to overcome the stigma is to put people at ease. Do this by speaking openly about the disease, and ask for help whenever you need it. That will help others overcome the fear and helplessness they feel when confronting Alzheimer's disease. ■

CONCLUSION

The authors are realists. We know that living with Alzheimer's disease is difficult. We also know that you can still have many wonderful and meaningful experiences, if you allow yourself to have them. We know patients who became world travelers, and others who grew very close to their families. A few continued to work for a while, then found great satisfaction from volunteering. They went to movies and plays, concerts and operas, walked in the woods and devoured barbecue with friends. Some have fought Alzheimer's disease by entering research and drug treatment programs. Patients have even written books about their experiences. One example is a fine book by Larry Rose called *Show Me The Way To Go Home*, published by Elder Books. Dale Thompson, one of the people to whom this book is dedicated, built a doll house for his granddaughters. He needed help, but it was his idea, he shared in the work, and his granddaughters loved it. We would not tell you that you could still enjoy your life, meet some goals, and be productive if we haven't seen others succeed in all these things.

Your next few years can be like this, *if you choose*. Anger and despair are easy mistakes to make. *You can refuse to be frustrated by the things that you can't do, and fully embrace all those things you can do.* Then all those movies, concerts, hikes, and dinners can be yours. If you want to be productive, and even fight Alzheimer's disease, that life can be yours as well. Grab it, live it, enjoy it!

Once you make that decision, you can prolong the best of your life by working to keep your body and mind in the best shape the disease allows. Exercise, eat well, fill your time with meaningful activity instead of frittering it away.

Do as much as you can for as long as possible. When something becomes frustrating, give it up and do other things instead. Do not be negative, and try not to be a wishful thinker. Be realistic about your capabilities.

Cover yourself legally. Maintain as much control over your financial and health decisions as possible by signing a durable power of attorney and a living will. Then you can rest in the knowledge that your intentions will be carried out if you are unable to make decisions later.

We know that making the best of the rest of your life can be challenging. There will be frustration and conflict. We also know these can be overcome if you commit yourself to live well. Don't be afraid to ask for help. Speak to social workers, lawyers, the Council on Aging, the Alzheimer's Association, and anyone else who can point you in the right direction.

The challenge to you is to enjoy the remaining years of your life. We know it can be done. We wish you all the best. ■

INDEX

A
abuse, 117
Acetyl-L-Carnitine, 13
activities, 71, 75
Adult Protective Services, 117, 118
age, 8, 12
alcohol, 39
Alzene, 13
anger, 53, 54, 57, 63, 83
anti-depressant medication, 85
anti-oxidants, 15
Aricept, 13
arts-and-crafts projects, 67
attitude, 6, 17
autobiography, 67
auto-immune abnormalities, 7

B
body changes, 94
bleeding, 15

C
calisthenics, 18
caregiver, 22, 53, 54, 57, 100, 102, 108, 110, 115
cash, 40
children, 11, 59, 109
chromosomal abnormalities, 7
cigarettes, 42
Cognex, 13
communication, 51, 83, 86, 88, 98, 100, 123
confusion, 82
conversation, 104, 105
cooking, 76
coping, 63, 69, 86

counseling, 55, 57, 60, 86, 87, 102
co-workers, 34, 36

D
daycare, 113, 114, 115
decisions, 98
depression, 80, 85, 87
DHEA, 13
diagnosis, 51, 90, 93
division of assets, 63
doctors, 90, 91, 93
drivers license, 45
driving, 45, 46, 47, 75
drug-testing programs, 30, 32
durable power of attorney, 53, 63, 116

E
Eldepryl, 14
embarrassment, 103
exercise, 17, 67, 85, 94, 122
experimental drugs, 13

F
family, 51, 55, 87, 103
family history, 8, 10, 12
fear, 11, 62
feelings, 86
finances, 41, 53, 76, 109, 115, 118, 119
fire, 76
free time, 67
friends, 61, 62, 103, 111
frustration, 71, 73, 83, 100, 102

G
genetics, 10
Ginkgo Biloba, 13
goals, 67, 69

H

health, 81
herbal remedies, 16
humor, 79, 80
hurt feelings, 99, 100, 102

I

Ibuprofen, 14
ID bracelet, 47, 49, 50
incontinence, 44, 90
itinerary of activities, 25

J

jigsaw puzzles, 67

L

laughter, 79
living trust, 53, 63
loneliness, 103
lost, 47, 49

M

major depressive disorder, 85
marriage, 54, 56
meaning in life, 65
Medic Alert bracelet, 47, 49, 50
medication, 13, 43, 72
memory, 70
mental stimulation, 18
Milameline, 14
mistakes, 34, 53, 76, 77
money, 40, 41, 115, 116, 118, 119
Motrin, 14
myoclonic movements, 94

N

neurotransmitter deficiencies, 7
NGF (Nerve Growth Factor), 14
Nimodipine, 14
nursing care, 115
nursing home, 108, 115, 121, 122

P

panic, 82
positive attitude, 17
prevention, 77

R

reactive depression, 85
reading, 28, 67
rejection, 62
research, 28
resentment, 54
respect, 66, 99
risk, 7, 11
role-reversal, 54, 59
rowing machine, 17
running, 17

S

Selegiline, 14
self-esteem, 37, 87
sex, 58
skills, 71
sleeplessness, 90
smell, 94
smoking, 42
socializing, 88, 103, 104
speech therapy, 107
spouse, 56, 121
stationary bicycle, 18

stigma, 125
stomach irritation, 15
strengths, 28
stress, 5, 6, 50, 64, 79, 82, 87
structured life, 23, 24
support group, 87, 88, 89, 103, 111
swimming, 18

T
tai-chi, 17
teenage children, 59
tests, 25, 26, 27, 28
transportation, 109
treatment, 13, 14
trust, 98

V
violence, 43
viral infections, 7
visual/spatial perception, 28
vitamin E, 14
vitamins, 15
volunteer work, 18, 33

W
walking, 17, 49, 67, 122
weaknesses, 28
weight loss, 94
word-finding, 106, 107
work, 33, 34, 35, 36, 37, 38

Appendix A
Useful Organizations

The following organizations provide information about Alzheimer's disease. Contact the National Alzheimer's Association and get on their newsletter mailing list. They may also be able to put you in contact with a local chapter and support group.

The Alzheimer's Association
919 North Michigan Avenue
Suite 1000
Chicago, IL 60611
1-800-272-3900   or   1-312-335-8700

National Institute of Mental Health
5600 Fisher's Lane, Rm. 7C02
Rockville, MD 20857
1-301-443-4513

Alzheimer's Disease Education and Referral Center
P.O. Box 8250
Silver Springs, MD 20907
1-800-438-4380
e-mail address: adear@alzheimers.org
Web-site: http://www.alzheimers.org/adear

APPENDIX B
SUGGESTED READING FOR PATIENTS

Rose, Larry. *Show Me The Way To Go Home*
CA: Elder Books, 1996

The author poignantly describes his painful experiences of living mid-life with Alzheimer's disease. He recalls the early signs and symptoms; the process of medical diagnosis and treatment; telling friends and family; coping with confusion, fear, and anger; and family involvement in decisions of property, caregiving, and support.

Friel, McGowin, Diana. *Living In The Labyrinth*
CA: Elder Books, 1993; NY: Dell Publishing, 1994

Writing in a simple direct style, the author describes her reactions to receiving a diagnosis of Alzheimer's disease and her experience of living with dementia. She relates both the innocent mistakes made and the successful positive steps taken in coping with this difficult and often overwhelming situation. Her message is one of hope and the importance of maintaining one's dignity and identity.

VIDEOS FOR PATIENTS

Alzheimer's Disease: Inside Looking Out
Chicago, IL: Terra Nova Films

This video shows individuals with early stage Alzheimer's discussing their experience with the disease, their feelings, and how they are coping.

A Thousand Tomorrows: Sexuality, Intimacy and Alzheimer's
Chicago, IL: Terra Nova Films

Interviews with spouses and individuals with Alzheimer's explore the effects of the disease on intimacy and sexuality in their relationship. It contains candid discussion of such issues as blurring of roles, changes in behavior that affect intimacy between partners, and sexual desire and attraction.

Early Onset Memory Loss — Conversations With Letty Tennis
Chicago, IL: Terra Nova Films

This video shows a woman in mid-life with early stage Alzheimer's attempting to cope with the changes the disease has brought on herself and her family. It helps dispel public misconceptions about people with memory impairing illnesses.

Suggested Reading For Caregivers

Davidson, Ann. *Alzheimer's: A Love Story*
NJ: Carol Publishing Group–A Birch Lane Press Book,
1997

In a series of fifty-six vignettes, each telling a complete story, the author provides an honest and moving description of life with an Alzheimer's patient. Progressing from the initial confusion and anger to a feeling of peace, she shares her experiences, beliefs, and emotions.

Mace, Nancy, L. and Rabins, Peter, V. *The 36 Hour Day*
New York: Warner Books 1992

Written especially for those caring for individuals with a dementing illness, the authors combine practical advice with specific examples and suggest constructive ways of dealing with the day-to-day stresses of caring for an impaired individual on a day-to-day basis. An excellent resource for anyone dealing with a dementing illness.

Caldwell, Marianne Dickerman. *Gone Without A Trace*
CA: Elder Books, 1995

Caldwell, a vocational nurse, poignantly reveals the personal journey she undertook when her 83-year old mother, who was suffering from Alzheimer's disease, quietly vanished from a New Hampshire neighborhood schoolyard in 1991. Factual information about Alzheimer's and the grieving process is combined with a unique "cookbook" recipe for the search process.

Sheridan, Carmel B. *Failure-Free Activities for the Alzheimer's Patient*, CA: Elder Books, 1987

The safe, reassuring activities in this book have many benefits — from letting the patient feel capable and involved to helping to keep the world from slipping away. From scrapbooks and music to outings, baking, and life collages, clearly illustrated instructions make each activity easy to do.

VIDEOS FOR CAREGIVERS

Living With Alzheimer's, Chicago, IL: Terra Nova Films

Designed for families and friends of newly diagnosed individuals, this video provides an excellent overview of how the disease affects the caregivers and families of those who have Alzheimer's disease.

Complaints of A Dutiful Daughter, Chicago, IL: Terra Nova Films

This video chronicles a daughter's response to her mother's illness, starting with the desire to cure and set things to right and progressing to eventual acceptance. Explores family relations, aging, change, and the meaning of love.

THE ALZHEIMER'S BOOKSHELF
P.O. Box 490 Forest Knolls CA 94933
1 800 909 COPE or 1 415 488 9002
Visit our website on the internet at:
http://www.nbn.com/~elder/alzheimer.html

ELDER BOOKS
Caring for Those Who Care

ORDER FORM

SEND TO:

Elder Books   Post Office Box 490   Forest Knolls CA 94933
PH: 1 800 909 COPE (2673)   FAX: 415 488 4720

PLEASE SEND ME:

Qty.	Title	Price/copy	Totals
____	*Alzheimer's: The Answers You Need*	@ *$10.95*	$_____.___
____	*In Sickness & in Health*	@ *$12.95*	$_____.___
____	*Show Me the Way to Go Home*	@ *$10.95*	$_____.___
____	*Gone Without A Trace*	@ *$10.95*	$_____.___
____	*Surviving Alzheimer's: A Guide for Families*	@ *$10.95*	$_____.___
____	*Failure-Free Activities*	@ *$10.95*	$_____.___
____	*Coping With Caring: Daily Reflections for Alzheimer's Caregivers*	@ *$11.95*	$_____.___

Total for books . . . .$_____.___

Total sales tax . . . . $_____.___

Total shipping . . . . $_____.___

Amount enclosed . . . . $_____.___

SHIPPING: $2.50 for first book, $1.25 for each additional book; California residents, please add 8.25% sales tax.

_____

Name

_____

Address

_____

City   State   Zip